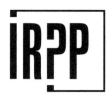

Institute for Research on Public Policy

Institut de recherche en politiques publiques

Founded in 1972, the Institute for Research on Public Policy is an independent, national, nonprofit organization.

IRPP seeks to improve public policy in Canada by generating research, providing insight and sparking debate that will contribute to the public policy decision-making process and strengthen the quality of the public policy decisions made by Canadian governments, citizens, institutions and organizations.

IRPP's independence is assured by an endowment fund established in the early 1970s.

Fondé en 1972, l'Institut de recherche en politiques publiques (IRPP) est un organisme canadien, indépendant et sans but lucratif.

L'IRPP cherche à améliorer les politiques publiques canadiennes en encourageant la recherche, en mettant de l'avant de nouvelles perspectives et en suscitant des débats qui contribueront au processus décisionnel en matière de politiques publiques et qui rehausseront la qualité des décisions que prennent les gouvernements, les citoyens, les institutions et les organismes canadiens.

L'indépendance de l'IRPP est assurée par un fonds de dotation établi au début des années 1970.

RIDING THE THIRD RAIL

THE STORY OF ONTARIO'S HEALTH SERVICES
RESTRUCTURING COMMISSION, 1996-2000

BY
DUNCAN SINCLAIR, MARK ROCHON AND PEGGY LEATT

THE INSTITUTE FOR RESEARCH ON PUBLIC POLICY

© The Institute for Research on Public Policy (IRPP)
2005
All rights reserved

Printed in Canada
Dépôt légal 2005

Library and Archives Canada
Bibliothèque nationale du Québec

Cataloguing in Publication

Sinclair, Duncan G.
Riding the third rail : the story of Ontario's Health
Services Restructuring Commission, 1996-2000 / by
Duncan Sinclair, Mark Rochon and Peggy Leatt.

Includes bibliographical references.
ISBN 0-88645-197-3

1. Ontario. Health Services Restructuring Commission.
2. Health care reform—Ontario. 3. Health planning—
Ontario. 4. Health services administration--Ontario.
I. Rochon, Mark II. Leatt, Peggy, 1940- III. Institute for
Research on Public Policy IV. Title.

RA395.C3S56 2005   362.1'09713   C2005-903860-8

PROJECT DIRECTORS
Hugh Segal and France St-Hilaire

EDITORIAL COORDINATOR
Francesca Worrall (IRPP)

COPY-EDITING
Jane Broderick

PROOFREADING
Mary Williams

COVER AND DESIGN
Schumacher Design

PRODUCTION COORDINATOR
Chantal Létourneau

PUBLISHED BY
Institute for Research on Public Policy (IRPP)
Institut de recherche en politiques publiques
1470 Peel Street, suite 200
Montreal, Quebec H3A 1T1
Tel: 514-985-2461
Fax: 514-985-2559
E-mail: irpp@irpp.org
www.irpp.org

To those who worked so hard to make change happen — commissioners, staff members and those "offstage" — and especially to Don Thornton, good colleague and friend departed.

CONTENTS

xii   LIST OF TABLES, FIGURES AND APPENDICES

xiii   LIST OF ABBREVIATIONS

xv   PUBLISHER'S NOTE

xvii   ACKNOWLEDGEMENTS

xix   FOREWORD

1   INTRODUCTION

9   **CHAPTER 1**
         ESTABLISHING THE HSRC
10   Historical Overview
17   Legislative Framework
19   The Establishment of the HSRC
30   Reactions

37   **CHAPTER 2**
         THE POLICY CONTEXT
42   The Need for Policy
45   Health Human Resources
49   Health Information Management
50   Aboriginal and Population Health
52   Mental Health
52   Home Care
54   Devolution
56   Initiatives Elsewhere

63	**CHAPTER 3**
	VOLUNTARY GOVERNANCE
68	Faith-Based Hospitals
71	Governance Models
76	Community Process
78	Lessons Learned
85	**CHAPTER 4**
	HOSPITAL RESTRUCTURING:
	THE COMMISSION'S POWER
89	District Health Council Reports
92	Health Information
93	Restructuring Methodology
100	Decision-Making Criteria
103	Results
105	Hospital Networks
106	Rural and Northern Hospitals
113	**CHAPTER 5**
	RECOMMENDATIONS LINKED TO HOSPITAL
	RESTRUCTURING: CONSTRAINTS ON POWER
118	Community Care Capacity
136	Action on Recommendations
141	**CHAPTER 6**
	THE RESTRUCTURING OF A
	HEALTH-SERVICES SYSTEM
144	Commission Retreat
144	Vision of the System
150	Public Opinion
150	Expert Advice on the Process of Change
152	Round-Table Discussions
153	Health Information Management
157	Primary Health Care
166	Improving Health System Performance through Greater Accountability
168	Integrating the System from the Ground Up
170	Academic Health Science Centres

175	**CHAPTER 7** **THE PUBLIC RELATIONS CHALLENGE**
191	**CHAPTER 8** **LEGAL CHALLENGES**
191	Sudbury General
193	Ontario Public Service Employees Union
194	Pembroke Civic
197	Wellesley Central Hospital and Doctors Hospital, Toronto
202	Hotel Dieu, Kingston
204	Douglas Memorial, Fort Erie
205	Montfort, Ottawa
208	Out-of-Court settlements
213	**CHAPTER 9** **WHAT HAPPENED, WHAT DIDN'T,** **WHAT'S NEXT**
225	What's Next?
229	**CHAPTER 10** **LESSONS LEARNED**
234	Conditions for Change
237	Local Leadership
239	Quantity/Quality
242	Communication
245	**CHAPTER 11** **IMPLICATIONS FOR PUBLIC POLICY**
248	Devolution
252	Getting Things Done
260	Barriers to Change
267	**AFTERWORD: TOWARD A GENUINE** **HEALTH CARE SYSTEM**
285	**BIBLIOGRAPHY**
289	**BIOGRAPHICAL NOTES**

LIST OF TABLES, FIGURES AND APPENDICES

Tables

- 98   Table 1
  Comparison of Acute-Care Beds in Place March 31, 2003, with HSRC Targets for 2003, by OHA Region and HSRC Grouping

- 129   Table 2
  Utilization of Long-Term-Care Services by Persons Aged 75 and Over

- 147   Table 3
  Essential Characteristics of a Genuinely Integrated Health System

Figures

- 12   Figure 1
  Changing Practice and Technology – Change in Surgical Activity and Acute Separations, 1989/90-1995/96

- 14   Figure 2
  Changing Practice and Technology – Hospital Beds Staffed and in Operation, 1989/90-1995/96

- 145   Figure 3
  Current and Future Models of Health Reform

- 146   Figure 4
  Integrated Health Systems

Appendices

- 33   Appendix 1
  Some Elements of Bill 26

- 80   Appendix 2
  Definitions of Governance Structures

- 82   Appendix 3
  HSRC-Appointed Governance Facilitators

- 172   Appendix 4
  Policy Forum Workshop Participants

ABBREVIATIONS

ALC	alternative level of care
CCAC	Community Care Access Centre
CHAO	Catholic Health Association of Ontario
CHC	Community Health Centre
CHM	Canada Health Monitor
CHST	Canada Health and Social Transfer
CIHI	Canadian Institute for Health Information
CT	computed tomography
DHC	District Health Council
DPG	Day-Procedure Group
EPF	Established Programs Financing
HSO	Health Service Organization
HSRC	Health Services Restructuring Commission
IAHS	Integrated Academic Health System
ICES	Institute for Clinical Evaluative Sciences
IHS	integrated heath system
JEC	Joint Executive Committee
LHIN	Local Health Integration Network
LTC	long-term care
MHA	Mental Health Agency
MHITF	Mental Health Implementation Task Force
MRI	magnetic resonance imaging
MTDHC	Metropolitan Toronto District Health Council
O and A	Orthopaedic and Arthritic Hospital
OCFP	Ontario College of Family Physicians
OMA	Ontario Medical Association
PCG	Primary Care Group
PPH	Provincial Psychiatric Hospital
RHA	regional health authority
RNAO	Registered Nurses Association of Ontario
TTH	the Toronto Hospital

PUBLISHER'S NOTE

Public policy is a mix of analysis, empirical research, political and philosophical direction and desired positive outcomes. That is the realm in which IRPP research usually operates, seeking wherever possible to strengthen the empirical knowledge about an issue that policy-makers are facing, in a way that constructively informs the decision-making process. That has been the Institute's mission since its founding in 1972.

Although *Riding the Third Rail: The Story of Ontario's Health Services Restructuring Commission, 1996-2000* deviates somewhat from normative empirical research, the IRPP is delighted to add it to the extensive work the Institute has done since 1997 on health care policy in Canada, because of the practical realities it so frankly and passionately describes.

Duncan Sinclair, Mark Rochon and Peggy Leatt have written a detailed account of the work of the Health Services Restructuring Commission, which was established on an arm's-length basis by the Harris government in Ontario in 1996. They are not dispassionate observers analyzing something others did twenty years ago, but individuals who, as commissioners or senior staff of the commission with a serious and challenging mandate for change conferred upon them by the Ontario government, put their lives and souls into the task. Their experiences, insights and frustrations will be important learning blocks for the ongoing implementation of health care reforms across Canada.

Governments are often accused of putting partisan politics ahead of objective public interest. The Health Services Restructuring Commission was established by the provincial government to ensure that the approach in sorting out appropriate priorities, changes, streamlining and reconfiguration around the service/institution matrix of health care delivery in Ontario was as objective as possible. The commission was given significant leeway and authority, and the individuals appointed to it were of outstanding caliber and experience. How it worked out and why presents a unique opportunity to learn about instruments of change in critical policy areas like health care.

The commission's work was not without controversy, and nor was the way the government addressed the decisions the commission made. All the more reason why this policy and operations memoire offers insights that will be invaluable to all who care about governance, health care, and how democracies achieve change in areas deeply influenced by stakeholder interests.

Hugh Segal
Montreal
May, 2005

ACKNOWLEDGEMENTS

As with most things, making change in health and health care is something that cannot be done alone; it is a team sport. This account describes the result of the individual efforts of many devoted men and women who together made up a remarkable team. Although we are unable to acknowledge the work of everyone, we sincerely appreciate and value each contribution, large and small, to all that Ontario's Health Services Restructuring Commission was able to achieve, from its inception in the late spring of 1996, through its sunset in 2000, to the end of its planning horizon in 2003.

We acknowledge particularly the dedicated work of the commissioners, volunteers all — Ruth Gallop, Shelly Jamieson, Harri Jansson, Maureen Law, Doug Lawson, George Lund, Hart MacDougall, Muriel Parent, Dan Ross, Don Thornton (deceased) and Rob Williams — who, together with their partners, cheerfully sacrificed enjoyable pursuits and countless hours to ensure that the commission's decisions and actions served the public interest. We include in their number George Pink, Sarah Rochon and Leona Sinclair, the last of whom took a four-year rain check on the start of shared retirement.

Special kudos go to those who made up the commission's staff — many at the start of their careers — hard-working, inventive, talented and imbued with infectious enthusiasm for the challenge of engaging in work with the potential to make a real difference. Each staff member made vital contributions but none more so than the team leaders, Peter Finkle and Mario Tino. We acknowledge especially the work of the commission's corporate secretary and general factotum, Beverly Nickoloff, without whose assistance, support and advice this book could not have been written.

Many other players contributed "offstage" to the HSRC's work. We acknowledge particularly the supportive roles of David Lindsay and Perry Martin; of the deputy ministers of health, especially Margaret Mottershead and later Sandy Lang and Jeff Lozon; and of Elizabeth Witmer, who served as minister during much of the commission's mandate. Invaluable to us were the direct participation of David Naylor as the HSRC established its modus operandi, the communications expertise of Bruce MacLellan, and the inspired guidance of John Laskin in finding paths through the legal thickets that threatened to entangle us.

We gratefully acknowledge the encouragement and financial support for the writing of this book received from the Ontario Hospital Association, the Canadian Health Services Research Foundation and the Faculty of Health Sciences of Queen's University.

To all who put a shoulder to the wheel, we extend our grateful thanks.

Duncan Sinclair
Mark Rochon
Peggy Leatt

FOREWORD

Our health system is filled with politics of a good and bad sort. At its best, politics energizes the formation of new public policy as the elected grapple with the reconciliation of old and new ways as well as the will of the electorate and the advice of experts. At its worst, politics mounts an ugly defence of the status quo and resistance to sensible change.

In undertaking one of the most important challenges in reforming Ontario's health system, the Health Services Restructuring Commission (HSRC) had plenty of both kinds of politics with which to contend. In restructuring hospitals and proposing a plan for integrated health services, the commission juxtaposed reason against politics and rationality against history. It proved to be an anything but easy task.

The HSRC represented a political decision to put at arms length the task of closing and amalgamating some Ontario hospitals. The commission was also charged with bringing forward a plan for health services and hospital services. At the core of the HSRC's work, and at the heart of *Riding the Third Rail: The Story of Ontario's Health Services Restructuring Commission, 1996-2000,* by Duncan Sinclair, the commission's chair, and Mark Rochon and Peggy Leatt, its two CEOs, is the essential and still incomplete task of transforming Canadian health services into a true system of care. This deceptively simple concept is our most daunting challenge since the advent of hospital insurance.

My own direct involvement with the work of the HSRC included work as a facilitator in two instances. I worked with the University Avenue hospitals, primarily the Toronto Hospital and Mount Sinai, to analyze the potential for better, more efficient services. That assignment led to program transfers among the hospitals, which strengthened hospital services. I also worked with Georgetown and District Hospital, Peel Memorial Hospital in Brampton, and Etobicoke Hospital to create the new multisite William Osler Health Centre. This successful merger was a tribute to the goodwill of everyone involved to achieve constructive change.

In all of my involvement with the HSRC, several things struck me forcefully. The first was the quality of the team: the determination and wisdom of Duncan Sinclair; the energy and insight of Mark Rochon, David Naylor, Peter

Finkle, Mario Tino and others; and the calm thoughtfulness of Peggy Leatt. Ontario's best and brightest in health care wrestled with these difficult decisions. I was also struck by the enormity and complexity of the task they faced.

The challenges in the two phases of the commission's work were vastly different. In restructuring hospitals, the HSRC had formal legal authority, and it exercised it to get the job done. The authors are clear that the Ontario government retained — through the powers of the purse — ultimate approval power. They are also direct and honest about the "deep frustration" of working with a government that failed to move decisively on the larger health service issues. Their recommendations on hospital restructuring were implemented, but those requiring government decisions to invest in community-based services were routinely ignored. On the broader and more important task of creating a real health care system out of the disparate elements, the HSRC had only the persuasive powers of insight and eloquence. In this volume, Sinclair, Rochon and Leatt have produced a rich, yet readable rendition of these two stories.

Riding the Third Rail: The Story of Ontario's Health Services Restructuring Commission, 1996-2000 is an example of one of the most promising developments in Canadian public policy in general and health care policy in particular: the occasional willingness of leaders of change management to share their experience and insights. The book reminded me that governments are often well served when they let experts play a role in tough decisions. Of special note is the afterword: "Toward a Genuine Health-Care System." As a state-of-the-union assessment, this survey of the current state of health reform is as good as it gets. Every Canadian, from the prime minister to the concerned citizen, would benefit from reading it. In particular, all those involved with the Local Health Integration networks should read this analysis with care. The book's final sentence, "Let's hope we can pick up the pace," is certainly a sentiment that is shared by millions of Canadians.

Michael B. Decter
Chair, Health Council of Canada
June 2005

INTRODUCTION

This is the story of Ontario's Health Services Restructuring Commission. Established in 1996, the commission (HSRC) was one of the first in a series of such bodies, provincial and federal, set up to find solutions to worsening problems in health care — principally resistance to change, painful cost containment and ineffective accountability. Preceded by the more cerebral National Forum on Health (1994-97), Ontario's HSRC (1996-2000) was followed in 2000 and 2001 by a series of provincial bodies in Quebec (Clair Commission), Saskatchewan (Fyke Commission) and Alberta (Mazankowski Council).[1] Subsequently the Standing Senate Committee on Social Affairs, Science and Technology (2002), chaired by Senator Michael Kirby, reported the results of its two-year study of the state of health care in Canada. Weeks later, sole commissioner Roy J. Romanow reported on the work of the Royal Commission on the Future of Health Care in Canada (2002). Canadian health care, provincially and nationally, does not want for study nor for well-informed advice on approaches to solving its problems.

Created with a four-year mandate by legislative authority in 1996, the HSRC differed from its successor provincial commissions and councils by virtue of its having the unprecedented and seemingly unconstrained authority to restructure public hospitals. This power of direction, binding on the hospitals affected, was coupled with the more conventional responsibility to recommend to the government, through the minister of health, other changes necessary to make the provision of health services in Ontario more efficient and effective.

The HSRC's 12 volunteer commissioners took their role as agents of change very seriously. Private citizens with widely differing backgrounds and experience, drawn from communities throughout Ontario, they worked hard and long. For much of the time they were exposed to the unaccustomed glare of media attention and sometimes to the vocal ire of people affected by their decisions. Their emolument of one dollar a year was well and truly earned.

The goal? To foster progress toward the development of a genuine, rational, health care *system* in which hospitals work efficiently both with one another and with all the other players that together provide the range of services needed by vulnerable people facing or experiencing risks to their health.

Did the commission succeed? Were the four years of toil worthwhile? Given the glacial pace of change in health care, a scant four years after the commission's "sunset" is too soon to say. Certainly the goal of an efficient and optimally effective health-services system[2] in Ontario or in any other province remains some way off.

But some progress has been made. As a direct result of the commission's work, many previously competing acute-care hospitals in most of the province's urban municipalities have been consolidated, allowing the new institutions to provide higher-quality services more cost-effectively. Investments have been made in the expansion of home-care services and the creation of more nursing-home places to accommodate hospitalized patients categorized as ALC (alternative level of care) — people who would be cared for better and less expensively somewhere other than in an acute-care hospital. Most importantly, perhaps, the HSRC broke the mould of the status quo ante; it used its power to demonstrate conclusively that structural and operational improvements *can* be made in the delivery of health services in Canada, even in cautious Ontario, where the iconic status of health care qualifies proposals for change as the political equivalent of the "third rail."

This account of the HSRC's work has been written by the three people closest to the action. Duncan Sinclair was chair of the commission for the full four years. Mark Rochon was its chief executive officer for the first two tumultuous years of hospital restructuring. Peggy Leatt served as CEO subsequently, during the increasingly uphill struggle to develop viable strategies for a government whose zest for change in health care policies was, by then, quickly eroding.

Although the ideal of cold objectivity has been kept front and centre throughout, the authors are keenly aware of how difficult it is to "see ourselves as others see us," to quote Robbie Burns. Therefore, caveat emptor! Others may interpret differently the motives, debates, decisions, events, results and reactions during and since the commission's life span, from April 1996 to March 2000. But this is the frank and unvarnished view of those who were at the centre of the action.

Why tell the story now? Although it is five years since the HSRC shut its doors, it is only two years since its planning horizon of 2003 was reached. Thus the results of its work can be considered current.

During its four-year mandate the commission:
> changed the landscape in 22 of Ontario's urban and regional communities by ordering amalgamations and "takeovers," creating larger hospital organizations capable of greater quality and economies of scale; closed

31 public, 6 private and 6 provincial psychiatric hospital sites, prompting major expansion, province-wide, in home care and facility-based long-term care
> articulated and publicized its vision of Ontario's future health care system as a series of interconnected, integrated, regional community-based health systems
> suggested ways and means of coordinating mental health services, region by region, and integrating them with other hospital- and community-based health and social services
> recommended the organization of small rural and northern hospitals into networks
> developed strategies to achieve (1) a capacity for effective health information management; (2) reform of primary health care; (3) integration of health services in communities committed to achieving it; (4) the capacity to measure and assess improvements in the performance of health care delivery and to enhance its productivity and accountability; (5) the establishment of academic health science networks; and (6) more effective governance, by the province, of the restructured health care system

As with seeds, some ideas germinate slowly, some erratically and others not at all. All must find fertile ground, water and warmth. When the commission completed its mandate we thought that telling its story immediately would do more harm than good. Candid description of still current events and debates could well have reinforced what we perceived then to be a backlash against the rapid change the HSRC had forced, particularly on hospitals. Exhaustion, brought on in part by the fast pace, took the form of growing resistance to change on the part of hospitals, other players and the government; resolve stiffened against even the idea of considering new ways of organizing the provision of health services.

Although we do not perceive the ground and climate to be any more welcoming of change now, four years on, it is improbable that the telling of the commission's story will have a negative effect on the halting progress of the reform of Ontario's health care system or, more accurately, the creation of a genuine health care system in Ontario. It may embolden some to take those safely-out-of-sight reports down from their dusty shelves to test the receptivity of new policy-makers and decision-makers to the ideas and strategies they contain. At the very least, students and observers of health care in Canada will have the opportunity to share, before they fade to fantasy, our recollections of a novel approach to reforming the way in which health services are organized and provided in Ontario and of an exhausting and tumultuous yet fascinating experience.

We begin with some history, if that is not too grand a term for such recent times, of the circumstances that applied in the mid-1990s, circumstances that led to the establishment of the HSRC with its unprecedented power to order the restructuring of Ontario's public hospitals. First we offer an explanation of why the newly elected government created the commission, thereby giving a small group of volunteers control over highly contentious decisions with the potential to affect, if not determine, that government's political future.

We then describe the HSRC's transformation from a legislative concept to a real entity with staff, an office, contracted consultants, various strategies, and, most importantly, a plan and schedule for tackling its mandate. Central to everything, of course, was the forging of relationships, with the minister and the Ministry of Health,[3] with hospitals and other organizations within the various health-provider communities, and, primarily through the media, with those members of the public who were keenly interested in and would be affected by our decisions.

We follow with a description of the policy context in which the commission was established — what was in place to guide its work and, more significantly, what was not. Centrally important was the HSRC's articulation of its vision of a genuine health-services system — how it would meet the needs of Ontarians into the twenty-first century. It was essential that this vision be complemented by a series of policy guidelines relating to the "sizing" of community-based services such as long-term and home care, to ensure that alternative kinds of care would be available to patients affected by the changes that the commission would make in the acute-care and other hospitals.

Although we would have preferred otherwise, our initial focus was hospital restructuring. Central to this work — phase I — was our understanding of voluntary governance. We devote a chapter to the strengths and weaknesses of this concept, and to how the HSRC approached and dealt with boards of directors that represented the communities served by Ontario's public hospitals and their legal owners. We then move on to hospital restructuring itself, the basic principles we applied, our approach, the difficulties we faced in dealing with both urban and rural hospitals, and the overall outcome. We include a number of specific examples as the story of phase I unfolds but have resisted the temptation to include a blow-by-blow account of our interactions with the various hospitals. This may be a disappointment to those looking for the "inside story" regarding their community and its hospitals, but that was never our intention in writing this book. Confidentiality was promised to those affected, and that promise has been kept.

Chapter 5 describes what constituted the HSRC's greatest frustration and worry — forging a better and timelier linkage between our binding directions to hospitals to change and action by the government to implement our recommendation for concomitant changes in other health services, principally investments in home and long-term care. That linkage, of course, constituted the government's constraint on the commission's legislated power to order hospital restructuring. We describe some of the difficulties we faced at our bureaucratic and political interfaces, how we and those on the opposing side dealt with them, and the outcomes that were achieved.

In chapter 6 we turn to phase II, the HSRC's second two years, during which it turned its attention to the development of recommendations to the government on how best to begin creating a health-services system out of what is colloquially referred to as a "field of silos." We discuss our analysis of why the system's many autonomous constituents — acute care; tertiary/quaternary care; academic medicine; continuing care; rehabilitation, psychiatric, specialty and other hospitals; family and specialist physicians; independent health facilities; home care; nursing homes (the list is a long one) remain so poorly coordinated. We describe our establishment of a priority order of strategies to foster greater collaboration and coordination among these many players in order to achieve greater continuity of care for patients and their families, who have little interest in institutional or professional autonomy.

Communication with the public and with hospitals and other health care providers was very important to the HSRC and to the achievement of our goals. We devote chapter 7 to the development and execution of a strategy to explain and "market" our work. We deal particularly with the role played by the media in describing to the general public the commission's role and responsibilities as well as the reasoning behind our decisions.

In chapter 8 we discuss what turned out to be our time-consuming involvement with the courts, often referred to within the commission as our "legal practice," where our directions to some hospitals were rigorously tested.

In chapter 9 we review things as we now see them, measured against the planning horizon of 2003, and offer advice on what might be done differently the next time a government responsible for the governance of health care turns to an arm's-length, apolitical body to do things that, for whatever reason, it cannot do itself. The lessons we learned during the HSRC's four-year mandate are set out in chapter 10 — what was accomplished, what was changed, what was and was not effective.

We conclude by analyzing the implications of the commission's work for public policy on health care in Canada and the lessons that policy-makers might learn from the experience. Here, we draw heavily on work done subsequent to the HSRC's sunset by provincial bodies in Quebec, Saskatchewan and Alberta, and nationally by Senators Kirby and colleagues and by Roy Romanow with his Royal Commission on the Future of Health Care in Canada, to demonstrate the broad consensus of expert opinion on how to proceed with the creation of a new policy framework to preserve and enhance what Canadians call medicare.

This, then, is the story of Ontario's Health Services Restructuring Commission as experienced from within.

NOTES

1. Commission d'étude sur les services de santé et les services sociaux (2000), Commission on Medicare (2000) and Premier's Advisory Council on Health (2001), respectively.
2. System is defined as a "complex whole, set of connected things or parts, organized body or material or immaterial things" (*The Concise Oxford Dictionary of Current English*, 1976).
3. During the commission's tenure, the name of the Ministry of Health was changed to the Ministry of Health and Long-Term Care.

CHAPTER 1

ESTABLISHING THE HSRC

Why was Ontario's Health Services Restructuring Commission created? To be blunt, the HSRC was created to deal with a set of problems that the government of Ontario and its senior bureaucrats believed they could not solve themselves except at very high political cost, particularly to the premier and the minister of health, the politicians at the point of the plough.

What problems? The most acute at the time was financial — a crisis caused by escalating expenditures in health care, coincident with very constrained tax revenues and a political imperative to quickly shrink Ontario's budgetary deficit. Within the health care funding envelope, the disproportionately great financial needs of hospitals were perceived to be crowding out the needs of other sectors, particularly home care and long-term care. This was coupled with the longstanding recognition that several Ontario cities had two or more hospitals in close proximity to one another that were competing to serve the same population in buildings that were half empty, badly depreciated and in dire need of capital renewal.

Changing circumstances attributable to a number of factors had long affected Ontario's hospitals, especially those providing acute care. Principal among the changes were those in medical technology and practice patterns leading to a marked shift from in-patient procedures to "in and out" surgery and other ambulatory services supported by community-care programs such as home care.

The most acute problems were, in fact, related not only to the fiscal crisis affecting hospitals but also to an urgent need to rebalance spending — to shift money away from hospitals to other sectors of the health care system that had to be strengthened in order to support the changing needs of patients and families and changing health care practices.

HISTORICAL OVERVIEW

To fully understand fully the attitude toward hospitals that prevailed in the mid-1990s one must go back 20 years. William Davis was premier, successor to George Drew, Leslie Frost and John Robarts, leaders of the Progressive Conservative dynasty that had held power in Ontario for 42 years. Frank Miller, the minister of health, decided that something had to be done about the fact that many of the province's increasingly costly urban acute-care hospitals were offering services that duplicated those provided by others in the same community, some just a stone's throw away. So he set about closing down those he considered supernumerary. A celebrated example was Doctors Hospital, situated in downtown Toronto almost adjacent to the much larger Toronto Western Hospital,[1] an institution with what most acknowledged to be much better facilities and a more qualified medical staff. There, for his pains, Miller was pelted with snowballs by protesting patients, staff and community members; the police had to rescue him from a mob. The resultant media furor was later linked to the fact that when Premier Miller (Frank Miller having succeeded Bill Davis as leader) went to the people, the Conservatives won by a narrow margin and quickly lost power. This short-lived minority government was succeeded by an alliance between the Liberals, led by David Peterson as premier, and the New Democrats, led by Bob Rae. In the next election the Liberals were victorious and formed a majority government. For current and aspiring politicians of all stripes — but especially Conservatives — the message was loud and clear: Mess with hospitals at your peril!

This message persisted through the two successive Liberal governments led by Peterson (1985-90) and Rae's New Democratic Party (NDP) government (1990-95), which followed. Clearly, it was still very much on the minds of the Conservatives when they were returned to power in 1995 with Mike Harris at the helm, flying their campaign flag — "the Common Sense Revolution."

That is not to say the Peterson and Rae governments did not try hard to create order in health care and control its big and rapidly growing appetite for money. Both premiers appointed health ministers drawn from among their most able, energetic and reform-minded colleagues. Both created and personally chaired councils[2] formed of influential and expert members of the public, backed up by high-powered staffs supporting vigorous research programs and the publication of well-argued proposals for reform. District Health Councils (DHCs), established some years previously by the Davis government as Ontario's toe-in-the-water test of regionalization of health care, were reinforced. These planning bodies were given mandates to advise on the most efficient and effective ways of providing the spectrum of health services, including hospital care, required in their various jurisdictions throughout the province.

In 1990 the redoubtable Elinor Caplan, minister of health in the second Peterson government, further tested the idea of regionalization, then in the process of being implemented elsewhere in Canada, by setting up the Southwestern Ontario Comprehensive Health System Planning Commission chaired by Earl Orser, a powerful and respected resident of London, Ontario. The Orser Commission was charged with developing a 10-year strategic plan for the control of health services in London and the southwestern region. Included in its recommendations was the commission's advocacy of a limited degree of devolution to the region.[3] Before its report was submitted, however, an election intervened. Peterson's Liberals were succeeded by Ontario's first-ever NDP government. Subsequently, the commission's report and its recommendation to devolve to the region substantial authority over hospital and other health services were shelved as the newcomers in Queen's Park scrambled to learn the ropes of governing a very large jurisdiction heading into a recession.

Throughout this whole period the growth of hospital funding continued to be constrained by all governments, budget by budget. The rate of increase in hospital costs, attributable primarily to wage and salary settlements coupled with the introduction of new technologies, was not matched by corresponding increases in revenue. Consequently, hospitals reduced their staffing levels and closed beds to avoid or at least limit deficit financing. The resultant decrease in capacity was offset by substantial growth in day surgery and a focus on reducing length of stay, a focus made possible by both the growing availability of new pharmaceutical agents and an expansion in home-care programs.

Late in the recession of the early 1990s the Rae government attempted to negotiate what it called a "social contract" with all public and quasi-public organizations and unions, including those representing hospital workers. In the end, it mandated what came to be known as "Rae Days," days off without pay that had the effect of sustaining employment levels but significantly reducing the wage bill throughout the broadly defined public sector, including in hospitals.

But when the Progressive Conservatives came to power in June 1995 hospitals were still consuming approximately 41 percent of the health budget of $17.8 billion. That health budget constituted 32 percent of the provincial budget, which itself included an operating deficit of $10 billion (Ontario Ministry of Finance 1995). During the preceding election campaign the Common Sense Revolution had committed the incoming government to eliminating that deficit, balancing the budget, paying down the provincial debt and, at the same time, reducing the tax burden on the electorate. Hospitals were identified as a prime target in the government's search for ways to reduce its spending.

Reducing the rate of growth of hospital funding, if not the total spent on hospitals, was one reason to put hospitals under the magnifying glass. But an even more compelling reason, especially for hospitals providing acute care, was the fact that new knowledge and technology had for years been making it possible to provide ambulatory patients with a wide range of services previously available only to admitted patients. This reason for scrutinizing hospitals applies still, and will probably do so into the foreseeable future. As illustrated in figure 1, surgical admissions were changing dramatically.

Figure 1
CHANGING PRACTICE AND TECHNOLOGY – CHANGE IN SURGICAL ACTIVITY AND ACUTE SEPARATIONS,[1] 1989/90 AND 1995/96

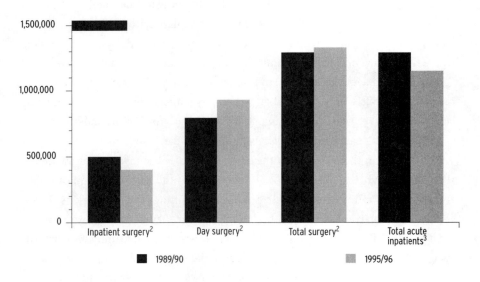

Source: Ontario Ministry of Health, Institutional Services Branch, 1996.
[1] Roughly equivalent to the number of people admitted to a hospital bed annually.
[2] Number of surgical admissions.
[3] Number of inpatient separations.

For example, whereas not long ago cataract surgery required patients to lie still in bed postoperatively for a week or two, their heads immobilized by sandbags, the procedure now rarely requires hospitalization, apart from the brief use of an operating room, and some question the need for even that. The development of minimally invasive "keyhole" surgery is another case in point; with the reduction in surgical trauma, many procedures that once required hospitalization can now be done safely on an ambulatory basis. The ever-growing panoply of pharmacological agents, the downside of which is the startling rate of growth in the share of health care spending on prescription drugs, means that people are now being treated for many conditions successfully and safely as outpatients. Similarly, modern diagnostic procedures and equipment continue to reduce the need for beds, especially in tertiary-care hospitals, the most costly of all hospitals.

For several years prior to the mid-1990s, international and interprovincial comparisons of the ratio of acute-care hospital beds to the served population provided a follow-the-leader rationale for governments to constrain the annual growth of their expenditures on hospitals. These comparative data created an incentive to constrain hospital funding even in jurisdictions, like Ontario, that were relatively quick off the mark in adjusting hospital in-patient capacity to reflect the changing balance between in-patient and outpatient procedures. According to an unpublished federal/provincial study,[4] in 1992-93 Ontario hospitals had one of the lowest average lengths of stay for acute care (seven days) and the lowest rate of utilization of acute-care services (694 patient days/1,000 population) when compared to hospitals in the rest of Canada. Between 1989-90 and 1993-94, according to data obtained from the Ontario Ministry of Health:

> average acute-care length of stay declined by 20 percent, from 8.2 to 7.0 days
> approximately 6,700 beds were closed (a decrease of 20 percent) (see figure 2)
> in-patient cases decreased by over 7 percent
> outpatient services increased by 6 percent

By 1996, when the HSRC was set up, the cumulative result was that Ontario's approximately 225 public hospitals held no fewer than between 9,000 and 11,000 empty (i.e., unstaffed) beds, the collected equivalent of 30 to 35 mid-sized hospitals. Although there had been discussions about ways to collaborate, and the odd partnership and merger[5] had taken place, not a single hospital had been closed. This was the case even in communities in which two institutions providing the same spectrum of services, sometimes but a short walk apart,

Figure 2
CHANGING PRACTICE AND TECHNOLOGY – HOSPITAL BEDS STAFFED AND IN OPERATION, 1989/90-1995/96

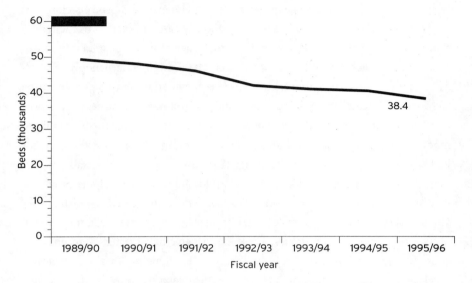

Source: Ontario Ministry of Health, Institutional Services Branch, 1996.

struggled to stay afloat and balance their books, each with empty wards and substantial numbers of patients in their remaining acute-care beds who did not require such intensive (and expensive) services.

The case for rationalization was obvious, particularly in cities with two or more public hospitals offering acute care. But memories of Frank Miller remained!

Toward the middle of the Rae government's term in office, Ruth Grier, Rae's third minister of health, called upon those DHCs whose jurisdictions included communities with more than one hospital to come up with recommendations on how best to reorganize the facilities and the spectrum of services they provided. The ultimate objective was more effective use of hospital resources and greater cooperation and collaboration both among hospitals and between hospitals and other health care providers.

The quality of and pace at which this work proceeded varied widely community by community. But it soon became apparent, from the very public nature of the discussions in which the participating DHCs engaged, that in no community or district would a clear consensus emerge for a plan to reduce the number of hospitals, regardless of the wealth of data and informed opinion marshalled to support it or the extent of community participation in the debate. In virtually all communities, winners and losers were identified (or identified themselves) early on. Camps were formed. During public consultations, opposing positions tended to become more deeply entrenched, even though the purpose of the public exercise was to produce outcomes that would minimize dissent. There were exceptions, however. In Windsor the DHC was remarkably successful in forging consensus on a hospital restructuring plan that incorporated some extremely hard decisions.

It was as clear to Grier's Tory successor as minister of health, Jim Wilson, as it had been to Grier that very few communities would be able to make the painful health care decisions needed, especially those related to reorganizing hospitals, their buildings and services. In some communities the DHCs had risen courageously and imaginatively to the challenge of openly scrutinizing the issues of quality, access, changing needs, costs and so forth.[6] They had produced well-argued reports that reflected both the wide range of options discussed in extensive public consultations and the rationale for their often unpopular recommendations. In other communities the DHCs did nothing but produce thick reports justifying, at great length, continuation of the status quo. In most affected communities it was clear that, independent of the strength of the evidence, public opinion remained divided and that local leadership was not strong enough to produce reports containing broad consensual decisions. In all affected communities, local leaders, no matter how courageous, needed substantial support from a central authority in order to proceed. Where genuinely hard decisions had been made, help with implementation of the locally developed plans was essential. "Somebody in Toronto" with authority to take action was going to have to provide that support.

And time was of the essence. The newly elected government had landed running. It was determined to use both the window of opportunity following its election and its large majority to implement the policies of the *Common Sense Revolution*. Although the recession of the early 1990s that had hammered the Rae government's agenda had eased somewhat, Ontario's manufacturing base was still recovering, tax revenues were predicted to increase very slowly over the near term and reduced federal transfers from Ottawa showed no sign of being restored, much less increasing. Despite the government's unwavering commitment to cutting taxes, its top priority was reducing the provincial deficit. The new government was determined to follow through on the campaign platform that had served so well to differentiate Mike Harris and his Conservatives from the challengers. This platform contained initiatives of the "short-term pain for long-term gain" variety based on the principle that if Ontario taxpayers had more money to spend, living standards and the economy would improve. In the meantime, government spending would have to be cut to fit tax revenues. The government had also made a very public commitment during the campaign not to get caught up in the politics of power and to be "true to its word" — not to deviate from the manifesto set out in the Common Sense Revolution.

So, early on, Premier Harris, his minister of finance, Ernie Eves, and the small cadre of influential elected and nonelected advisers who had crafted the campaign strategy focused on the big spenders among the government departments. Obviously, the Ministry of Health topped the list; equally obvious, within that ministry's spending envelope was the 41 percent ($17.8 billion) being consumed by hospitals. This was coupled with DHC reports of empty beds everywhere and comparative data from some other jurisdictions that showed Ontario, even discounting its 9,000 to 11,000 empty beds, had ample capacity to meet its population's need for acute-care services, provided that its hospitals' ALC (alternative level of care) patients could be cared for elsewhere. There was also a need to acknowledge publicly the change in the nature of health care — the shift from hospital to ambulatory care and the need for improved coordination among hospitals and between hospitals and other providers of care, to keep people from falling through the cracks. Without improved system planning and coordination among all providers, continued across-the-board cuts would jeopardize both the quality of hospital services and the ability of home and community services to respond to the inexorable pressures being placed on them by the changes in service delivery.

In 1995 this already unstable environment was rocked by two announcements made by a very new government. The good news was that the total funding of health care by the Ministry of Health would not be reduced; it would remain stable throughout the life of the government. The bad news was that the budget for hospitals would be reduced by 18 percent over three years, at the rate of 5 percent in 1996-97, 6 percent in 1997-98 and 7 percent[7] in 1998-99. This response reflected the government's view that cost saving in hospitals represented "low-hanging fruit" relative to such issues as the physicians' fee schedule, physician productivity or the job descriptions of health professionals as set by the various guilds.

What passes for wisdom in health care politics is a reluctance to open up too many fronts at a time. So the conclusion was that priority should be given to "restructuring" public hospitals, a word and concept then au courant in the management literature. But how to do this? The lesson of the unhappy experience of Frank Miller, then still living in a community not far from the ridings represented by Premier Harris and the Honourable Mr. Eves, was deeply ingrained.

The members of the HSRC were not privy, of course, to the in-camera discussions that led to the decision to establish an arm's-length commission and have it do the deed. Nor were they subsequently told whose idea this was, who was for and against, and how the argument went in relation to the key question of if, how and to what degree the government could be insulated from the political consequences of the commission's decisions. Those matters remain cloaked in the secrecy accorded cabinet discussions.

LEGISLATIVE FRAMEWORK

Although the *Public Hospitals Act*, the *Ministry of Health Act* and other legislative instruments, with their attendant regulations, have long been in place to link public policy and its application, it is fair to say that, at the time of the HSRC's appointment, past practice and ministerial policy directives predominated in defining the relationship between hospitals and the government. The submission of budgets and annual reporting on hospital activities, services and related expenditures were responsibilities codified and directed by officials in the health ministry acting on the authority of the minister. Advice to this policy process originates in many places, but since 1992 prime responsibility has rested with the Joint Planning and Policy Committee. This body was set up by the ministry and the Ontario Hospital Association to maintain the currency of policy and practices with contemporary and anticipated circumstances affecting hospitals. This somewhat fluid, evolutionary approach to government supervision of the work of hospitals throughout the province developed as an alternative to periodically updating the now somewhat antiquated legislative framework.

The statutory and regulatory framework within which hospitals operate dates back to the 1930s.[8] Although the *Public Hospitals Act* was intensively reviewed in the early 1990s with a view to bringing it up to date, it has remained as written originally, amended only in the early 1980s to allow for the appointment of investigators and supervisors in the event of a hospital's failing to discharge its responsibilities to the minister's satisfaction. The *Public Hospitals Act* and associated legislation, including the *Ministry of Health Act,* give the government spending and other regulatory authority that has long been considered sufficient to provide it with the power needed to ensure that hospitals meet the goals of public policy.

Given the task of hospital restructuring foreseen in 1995, however, the Harris government was concerned that the existing statutory framework did not provide it with sufficient authority to make the contemplated changes. Accordingly it introduced Bill 26, the *Savings and Restructuring Act.* The opposition parties argued that the "draconian measures" suggested in this bill, introduced during the November 1995 Economic Statement, were unnecessary because, through normal allocative processes, the "power of the purse" gave the government a tool sufficient to achieve its ends. The government and its advisers were of the view that the outcomes contemplated required measures beyond what could be achieved by simply turning on the money tap. They believed that greater authority was needed to give government the explicit power to shut hospitals down. As shown subsequently in judicial rulings made following challenges to the HSRC's directions, the government was right.

The great majority of hospitals in Ontario are not "public" in the sense of being publicly owned and operated. Nearly all are private institutions, answerable, like other private entities, to boards of directors representing the federally or provincially registered corporations that own them. That virtually all of those corporations are charitable and operate on a not-for-profit basis is beside the point. Legally they cannot be ordered around as if they were part of a government department. Hospitals are considered public institutions because, of course, their services are available to the public and the great majority of their funding comes from the public purse. So defined, they are required to be in good standing with the government of the day, acting through the minister of health and his or her officials in the ministry. Basically, hospitals can be thought of collectively as privately owned and operated institutions acting as a regulated public utility.

THE ESTABLISHMENT OF THE HSRC

On November 29, 1995, Bill 26 (the *Savings and Restructuring Act*) received first reading in the legislature (see appendix 1). This was an omnibus bill proposing amendments to more than 40 pieces of provincial legislation, notably, with respect to health care and the work of the HSRC, acts applying to the Ministries of Health and Municipal Affairs and the Treasury. The Bill's purpose was to achieve fiscal savings and promote economic prosperity through public-sector restructuring, streamlining and more efficient operation.

The commission's mandate flowed from legislation affected by Bill 26 and from regulations issued subsequently under the *Ministry of Health Act* and the *Public Hospitals Act*[9] as amended. Schedule F of Bill 26 amended the requisite health-services acts[10] and created the HSRC, "sunsetting" it after four years.

The minister of health was given sweeping powers to reorganize health care by, for example, restructuring public hospitals, reducing or terminating grants or loans and ordering the boards of public hospitals to close, amalgamate, or provide or cease to provide specified services. By direction, the minister could also revoke the licence of a private hospital and reduce or terminate its funding. Upon the recommendation of the minister, the Lieutenant-Governor in Council could replace a hospital board with a supervisor to ensure compliance with directions. Finally, the minister was authorized to delegate his or her direction-making powers to other bodies — and this is where the HSRC came in.

Barring additional legislative action, Bill 26 provided for the expiry of most of these powers on March 1, 2000, four years after the enabling section of Bill 26 came into force, although it also provided that directions issued pursuant to them would retain the force of law. Regulations[11] gave the commission the authority to issue binding directions to hospitals. They did not confer any authority over the unions representing their workers; their cooperation could not be compelled. Practically speaking, such cooperation can be assured only when unions consider it in the best interests of their members. Neither could the commission commit the government to spend money. In addition, while the commission could, by direction, bind public hospitals to take specified actions, it could only advise the minister with respect to the province's psychiatric hospitals and/or on issues related to reinvestments and other changes required to support restructuring.

While legally established at arm's length from government, the commission was authorized to function in accordance with the government's fiscal and other policies. It was to be accountable to the minister of health in respect of its duties and powers. The legislation made it clear, however, that the commission could make independent decisions on hospital restructuring; these did not require the minister's concurrence.

After a raucous and occasionally rancorous debate on what the opposition dubbed the "Bully Bill," Bill 26 was passed and given Royal Assent on January 30, 1996.[12]

Nothing comparable to this piece of legislation, giving the HSRC what amounted to the power of the government itself over hospitals, has ever been enacted in a Canadian province. Although the details of its origins remain behind the veil of cabinet secrecy, the idea for Bill 26 was embedded within the restructuring report of the Metropolitan Toronto District Health Council. Released in September 1995, the report recommended the closure or merger of a dozen of Metro's 44 hospitals and the creation of a body to oversee the process (Metropolitan Toronto District Health Council 1995). Although the commissioners themselves were unable to verify this, it was said at the time that there was a precedent in the United States in the form of the Base Closure and Realignment Commission, a body given power by both the president and Congress to rationalize a perceived superfluity of military bases after the end of the Cold War.[13]

Whether the American precedent existed or not, the power given to the HSRC — to order hospitals to amalgamate, transfer or accept programs, change the focus of their work or cease to operate, or to make any other change considered to be in the public interest — was from the outset and is still considered in Canada and internationally as both unique and unprecedented. Nowhere else has a government delegated so much power over such a politically sensitive field of endeavour as health care provided in and by hospitals. Not surprisingly, this provision captured the attention of opposition politicians (and of some on the government bench), the media, and particularly hospital board members and their supporters, hospital unions and hospital employees. It presented the commission with the ongoing communications challenge of reminding anyone who would listen that the HSRC was the *Health Services* Restructuring Commission, not the *Hospital* Restructuring Commission. The distinction was an important one, especially for the commissioners, for whom hospital restructuring was, from the outset, an unpleasant, difficult, time-consuming and very public but necessary step toward the goal of a more coordinated and genuine province-wide health care system.

Ontario was the last province to approach hospital rationalization in the 1990s. It also chose to use a mechanism different from devolution to regional health authorities (RHAs) used by the other provinces. Instead it established the HSRC, a province-wide, arm's-length commission with a limited term, to determine what was necessary and exercise the power to have it done.

In the 1990s most of the other provinces[14] partially devolved their responsibility for health care delivery to subprovincial regions or RHAs. In fact, decentralization of authority and accountability for health services has been a strategy used in every province except Ontario. The move toward regionalization was driven by a desire to rid health care of its "silos" and to improve access to high-quality care at reasonable cost. Under these structures, typically a provincially appointed[15] board is accountable to the province/territory, through its ministry of health, for the delivery of a spectrum of health services and programs to the people of the region, paid for by government. The scope of institutional and community services managed and delivered by RHAs varies by jurisdiction (Standing Senate Committee 2002b, 65).

For the most part, however, RHAs, even those with responsibilities that extend across many institutions and service providers, have found it impossible to eliminate the silos and difficult issues related to excess institutional service capacity. There are examples of consolidation and successful role redefinition in some provinces; however, local politics and the notions of "fair share" that come into play when one regional jurisdiction is compared with another have often got in the way of local decision-making, just as they have when decisions of this nature have been attempted centrally by governments.

Many jurisdictions that established RHAs have had some success, however, in reducing administrative costs. For example, prior to regionalization Alberta had over 150 independent organizations, each with its own board and rank of senior managers, whereas now it has nine RHAs.[16] Savings have also been achieved in "back office" costs such as supplies, financial services, human resources and purchasing. However, efficiencies achieved through horizontal integration of community services and vertical integration of community and institution services are rare: "Although boards have integrated and rationalized parts of the institutional sector, integration of the community sector is hampered by structural constraints such as the lack of budgetary authority for a broader scope of services, including physicians' fees and drugs" (Lomas 1997).

The HSRC's formal mandate was to undertake three interrelated tasks:
> to make binding decisions on the restructuring of public hospitals
> to make recommendations to the government, through the minister of health, on the restructuring of other sectors or elements providing health services, including on reinvestments needed to support hospital restructuring and to enhance the provision of other health services
> to foster the creation of a genuinely integrated, coordinated health care system

This mandate proved to be cleverly constructed, especially with regard to the linkage between the power to make binding decisions regarding hospitals and the authority only to make recommendations on the restructuring of everything else. Any major changes affecting the hospital sector will, of course, inevitably produce consequences for other providers of health care, especially home care and long-term care. If those other providers are not prepared and funded to meet these consequences, primarily the care of patients discharged from acute-care beds, hospital restructuring is blocked. So, in the end, although the commission's unprecedented power appeared to be absolute, unfettered by political or other influences and decisions and binding on the government, in fact the government continued to be very much in control. It held the trump card by virtue of its right to decide what, if any, action to take on the commission's recommendations related to the reinvestments needed to support hospital restructuring and its advice on restructuring other sectors of health care.

Was the commission truly independent of government? Yes — with respect to the decisions bearing on hospitals individually. But it was entirely dependent on government with respect to implementation of its recommendations on hospital restructuring, both generally and community by community. If its advice to reinvest in community-based home care and long-term care was not taken, hospital restructuring was effectively blocked by the spectre of vulnerable people being put on the street, something the commission refused to countenance. It said so publicly, explicitly and repeatedly.

At the outset and throughout its four-year term, the commission's third task, fostering the creation of a genuinely integrated, coordinated health care system, received the least attention from government, health care providers, the media and the public. Yet this was the touchstone that caught the imagination of the commissioners from the outset, primarily because it had the greatest potential to benefit the system and the people it serves. It was the system-building challenge that was uppermost in the decision of most if not all of the commissioners to join an enterprise they knew from the start would win them few friends and likely create an enemy or two.

Notwithstanding all the frequent references to a health care system, no province, nor Canada as a whole, has one, if we take the word *system* to mean an organization in which the many different and diverse parts function together. Tommy Douglas observed that it had been his and his fellow pioneers' intention from the outset to create Medicare in two steps. The first was to remove the financial barrier between those who needed health care and those who provided it. Care was defined in those days as in-hospital care and somewhat later also as care by physicians. That step led to the adoption by all provinces of publicly funded health care insurance plans that adhere to the five famous principles of the *Canada Health Act:* universality, accessibility, portability, comprehensiveness and public, not-for-profit administration of the insurance plans themselves. The second step, which the Honourable Mr. Douglas wryly observed in 1982 had yet to be taken, was to reorganize the provision of health care into a genuine system to optimize the effectiveness and efficiency of delivery and provide those it serves with continuity of care and taxpayers with the benefits of a real system's synergy: "When we began to plan Medicare, we pointed out that it would be in two phases. The first phase would be to remove the financial barrier between those giving the service and those receiving it. The second phase would be to reorganize and revamp the delivery system — and, of course, that's the big item. It's the big thing we haven't done yet" (Decter 1994, 14).

We still haven't done it! It was advancing the course of coordinated health services and creating a genuine health care system that the commission considered its greatest challenge — an opportunity to make a difference to health care in Ontario and Canada. How to take Premier Douglas's second step has been the focus of the work of other provincial commissions[17] and, most recently, the Standing Senate Committee on Social Affairs, Science and Technology (200a, b) and the Royal Commission on the Future of Health Care in Canada (2002).

That focus explains the HSRC's insistence that it was not the *Hospital* Restructuring Commission despite the widespread belief that it had the power to restructure hospitals. It was this narrow part of the HSRC's mandate that attracted and held media and public attention throughout its four-year term. It was a communications challenge to direct the attention of anyone who would listen to the much more important goal of organizing the "field of silos" that provide health services in Ontario into a genuine health care system.

Who were the commissioners? How were they appointed, and by whom? Appointments were made by the Ontario cabinet; each appointment was subject to an individual order-in-council. The commission's life began in February 1996 with the appointment of the chair, Duncan Sinclair, a physiologist soon to retire after completing a second term as dean of medicine and vice-principal of health sciences at Queen's University in Kingston. Previously he had chaired the research committee of Premier Rae's Council on Health, Well-Being and Social Justice and before that the governance subcommittee of Elinor Caplan's committee to review the *Public Hospitals Act*. He had served on the Orser Commission, was a member of the board of the Ontario Cancer Treatment and Research Foundation and had chaired a working group on human resources planning for the Provincial Cancer Network, the forerunner of Cancer Care Ontario. At the time of his appointment he was also a member of the National Forum on Health.

The process of Sinclair's appointment began in late 1995 at a meeting with Margaret Mottershead, deputy minister of health; the meeting concerned a novel alternative funding plan recently negotiated with the ministry and implemented in the Queen's Faculty of Medicine. Under this plan the Faculty of Medicine undertook full responsibility for recompensing its clinical staff for their comprehensive teaching, research, administrative and clinical responsibilities; their fee-for-service billings to the Ontario Health Insurance Plan ceased. At the end of the meeting Mottershead shared the confidence that the government was considering establishing a "high level" body to examine health care in Ontario and asked, "Would you be willing to consider serving on such a body?" Sinclair, wondering what could be added to the work of the then-current National Forum on Health and the two successive Premier's Councils, nevertheless said that, if asked, he would be pleased to consider it. When they met a couple of weeks later, Mottershead broached the idea of Sinclair's chairing what was at that stage a rather nebulous high-level body. He told her that he would agree to participate as a member but not as chair; he and his wife were looking forward to more free time and fewer responsibilities upon his retirement six months hence. Shortly thereafter Sinclair became aware of the continuing involvement of David Naylor in the concept. Naylor, a physician, was executive director of the Institute for Clinical Evaluative Sciences (ICES) (now dean of medicine and president-elect of the University of Toronto) and an insightful thinker on health care reform in Canada and internationally. After a number of conversations with Mottershead and Naylor, Sinclair agreed to accept the role of chair, if and when asked by the premier, at a meeting with Mottershead and Naylor during which the mandate and powers of the putative commission were fleshed out.

Sinclair was persuaded by three factors. The proposed body represented an opportunity to break out of the endless cycle of discussions and take action on some of the recommendations contained in the many excellent reports on health care languishing in the offices of government officials and health care providers across Ontario, throughout Canada and elsewhere. Sinclair also wished to spare his young friend Naylor for the other challenges to which he seemed destined. And finally, Sinclair considered it his duty to his grandchildren and their generation to ensure that Ontario's health care system would be there to provide first-class service if and when they needed it.

After his appointment in February 1995, Sinclair was a very busy man, getting the commission up and running while completing his term as dean of medicine. A major challenge was to prepare to hand over to his successor the running of the faculty and its novel alternative funding plan, with its new supporting organization, the Southeastern Academic Medical Organization. His agreement to chair the commission marked the start of the most harried and hectic four months of Sinclair's life.

A key task was to identify and submit, for the government's consideration, the names of well-qualified people to serve on the commission.

Six commissioners were appointed in March:
> Shelly Jamieson, Toronto-based executive director of the Ontario Nursing Home Association who subsequently, during the commission's term, was appointed executive vice-president of Extendicare (Canada) Incorporated. A former consultant in long-term care with broad knowledge of the care continuum, she had particular experience with the provision of community-based long-term care by both the public and private sectors. Jamieson was past chair of the Ontario Health Providers' Alliance, a group of 19 associations committed to ensuring a viable future for Ontario's health care system.
> Maureen Law, a former federal deputy minister of health and director general for health sciences of the International Development Research Centre, who during the commission's mandate became director of health, nutrition and population for the East Asia region of the World Bank in Washington. A physician who once served as deputy medical officer of health for York

County, Law had extensive experience in the federal department of health and welfare and in international health, including service as chair of the World Health Organization and as a member of its Global Commissions on AIDS and on Women's Health.
> George Lund, president and chief executive officer of Baton Broadcasting Systems of Northern Ontario, became a senior vice-president of the CTV television network during the commission's term. Originally from Alberta, resident in Sudbury since 1962, Lund had served on Sudbury City Council and in 1980 was elected chair of the Sudbury Regional Municipality. Founding president of Science North, he also served on the board of Algoma Hospital for a number of years.
> Hartland MacDougall, a career banker soon to retire as deputy chair of London Life, had previously been vice-chair of the Bank of Montreal and chair of Royal Trust. Founding chair of the St. Michael's Hospital Foundation, the Japan Society and Heritage Canada, MacDougall also chaired the Canada Japan Business Committee, the Council for Canadian Unity and the International Council for the Duke of Edinburgh Awards. Throughout his career he had served on a number of hospital boards and with a variety of health care organizations across Canada.
> Dan Ross, a London-based lawyer and a managing partner in the firm of McCarthy, Tétrault. Experienced in health care matters, Ross was a member of the merger task force that reorganized London's Victoria and University hospitals as well as past chair of the London Health Science Centre Foundation and a member of its board and executive committee.
> Don Thornton of Oshawa was a retired General Motors Canada executive with extensive background in business and financial management and experience with re-engineering and restructuring. He had served on the board of the Oshawa General Hospital for 15 years, including a term as chair, and on the hospital's foundation. Experienced in the voluntary and not-for-profit sector, Thornton was also past chair of the Oshawa Harbour Commission and a member of the Parkwood Foundation, the Canadian Chamber of Commerce and the Financial Executives Institute.

This core group of founding commissioners held their first meeting on April 24, 1996, shortly after the appointment by the chair of Mark Rochon as chief executive officer, Beverly Nickoloff as secretary (and, at that stage, doer-of-all-work) and David Naylor as special adviser to the chair.

At the time of his appointment, Rochon had been president and chief executive officer of Humber Memorial Hospital for six years and, previously, executive director of Georgetown Memorial Hospital. He and Sinclair had served together on the steering committee for review of the *Public Hospitals Act*[18] and its Governance Task Force; in 1994-95 he had been seconded to the Ontario Ministry of Health, serving as assistant deputy minister of institutional health with primary responsibility for hospitals.

An experienced public servant working in the Ministry of Health, Nickoloff had most recently served on the staff of the Premier's Council on Health, Well-Being and Social Justice, where she also worked with Sinclair while providing support to a number of its policy committees. She had long experience in government, including a stint (1983-85) on the political staff of the minister of health.

Naylor served as special adviser to the chair and HSRC until March 1998. A practising physician and an international expert on health services research, he brought to the commission a particular perspective gained from his analyses of variations in the rates at which hospital-based and other services are provided in different parts of Ontario; these analyses were incorporated in the province's first practice atlas, published by ICES.

Recognizing the need to proceed apace, the commission met 12 times between April and the end of December 1996. It quickly realized that more members were needed if it was to deal with a busy schedule of community-by-community hospital reviews and assign two of its members to each community as lead and associate commissioners. In response to a request by the chair, five more members were appointed.

> Doug Lawson, a senior partner in the McTague law firm in Windsor, was appointed later in 1996. One-time president of the Ontario Chamber of Commerce and founding chair of the Association of District Health Councils of Ontario, Lawson had served on the Orser Commission and as chair of the Cardiac Care Network Task Force. In addition, he had been instrumental in the merger of two hospitals, the Metropolitan General and the Windsor Western (now the Windsor Regional Hospital).

Three members were added in April 1997:

> Harri Jansson, an executive vice-president of the Bank of Montreal, had served as chair of the Vancouver General Hospital Foundation and on the boards of St. Boniface General Hospital in Winnipeg and Sunnybrook Hospital Foundation in Toronto. He was a member of the Canadian

Bankers' Association (Ontario Committee) and the Regional Board of the Institute of Canadian Bankers and was a director of Kids Help Phone and the Commonwealth Centre for Sports Development. Jansson resigned from the commission in March 1998, when he moved to Vancouver to become president and chief executive officer of Richmond Savings.

> Muriel Parent, a francophone former school and community college teacher from Val Rita in northern Ontario, was president and chief executive officer of a trucking company and two other family businesses. A committed advocate for and participant in her community, in addition to serving on the board of directors of the Sensenbrenner Hospital and the boards of management for the Cochrane District Homes for the Aged and the North Cochrane Children's Aid Society, Parent had served as reeve of the Corporation of Val Rita-Harty.

> Rob Williams, a family physician and chief of staff of the Timmins and District General Hospital, had co-authored an Ontario Medical Association (OMA) 1996 position paper, *The Physician's Role in Hospital Restructuring*. Williams had a long record of participation in professional and health care organizations, including the OMA's Committee on Hospitals and the Utilization Steering Committee of its Joint Planning and Policy Committee, as well as the Canadian Institute for Health Information Physician Advisory Group. He was an active promoter of and participant in telemedicine in the province.

The last member of the HSRC was appointed in the fall of 1998.

> Ruth Gallop, professor and associate dean of research in the Faculty of Nursing of the University of Toronto, also held appointments in the university's Department of Psychiatry and Division of Women's Mental Health. A long-time member of the advisory board of Ontario's Psychiatric Patient Advisory Office, she brought to the commission many years of nursing experience, particularly in mental health services.

It was important that the commission be relatively small so that its members could debate and work together as a team, avoiding camps and the spectre of some being (or perceived as being) "captured" by any particular interest group. Yet it was also vital that the commissioners have different backgrounds and experience and a collective sense of the diversity of Ontario, urban and rural, southern and northern, big city and small. Although settling on fewer than a dozen members imposed a heavy workload on each, the mutual respect and coherence that was quickly established among them justified the trade-off, measured in terms of both the fast pace set from the beginning and the pleasure and sense of commitment and satisfaction the commissioners took from their work together.

Not all potential appointees agreed or were able to serve on the commission. Some people approached by Sinclair declined because they could not, in good conscience, take on the heavy workload in addition to their other responsibilities. The employer of one knowledgeable, experienced and willing prospective member in northwestern Ontario denied a request for the flexible work schedule necessary to accommodate her responsibilities as a commissioner.

The commission's cast of ex officio members was complete in September 1998 when Peggy Leatt was appointed chief executive officer following Mark Rochon's resignation to take up the position of president and chief executive officer of the Toronto Rehabilitation Institute. Leatt had just completed the second of two five-year terms as chair of the University of Toronto's Department of Health Administration.[19] Author of many publications on health policy and health-services design and restructuring, Leatt, now professor and chair of the prestigious Department of Health Policy and Administration in the University of North Carolina's School of Public Health, is a widely recognized and respected expert on issues related to organizational behaviour and design.

The commissioners brought to their deliberations different perspectives from their varied backgrounds and experience. But all shared the commitment to use the opportunity presented by the HSRC to make changes in Ontario's hospitals and health care that would serve the public interest into a future that would be very different from the present or the past. They volunteered their expertise and considerable time and energy to the cause of public service. They certainly did not do it for the money; each was paid an honorarium of one dollar per year for the many hours spent deliberating in meetings, making hard decisions, visiting communities as lead or associate commissioner, giving interviews, examining data and poring over documents.

All strong-minded individuals, the commissioners frequently engaged in vigorous debate. Beginning from widely divergent positions, the debates almost always resulted in consensus on the course of action that was wisest and best served the public interest. Whether reached by consensus or — occasionally, on particularly contentious issues — by vote, decisions were invariably supported fully and unreservedly by all commissioners. None had taken on the role of commissioner for self-aggrandizement. The decisions of the commission would draw the type of reaction that had more potential to tarnish than to enhance reputations. The members' dedication was in the best tradition of public service.

REACTIONS

Reactions to the formation of the HSRC were surprisingly muted. They varied according to constituency. Although the opposition parties in the legislature argued vehemently and voted against Bill 26, once it passed they, like the governing party's caucus and supporters, appeared to accept the commission as a reasonable way of proceeding with the difficult but necessary task of restructuring hospitals and health care in general. The commission's chair and chief executive officer both issued a standing offer to attend any caucus or other meeting called by any party to discuss the work of the HSRC. Subsequently meetings were held with the Conservative caucus prior to the election in 1998, and with the Liberal caucus later on.

The most negative reaction came from the several unions representing hospital workers. The *Savings and Restructuring Act,* under which the commission functioned, made changes to labour legislation that were perceived to have the effect of diminishing union power. Surprisingly, however, the expression of that negative reaction was relatively mild and did not last long after the Act was passed and the commission established. The unions affected were far more concerned with what they viewed as the Conservative government's negative attitude toward organized labour in general. They objected strenuously to its announced intention to shrink the size and activities of the government and its civil service. The government's implementation of that strategy was a problem for the public-sector unions in the spring of 1996, whereas the commission merely represented a problem likely to come later when its decisions began to appear.

The reaction of the Ontario Hospital Association was mixed. Many of the teaching and large urban hospitals that provided the greatest range of sophisticated services tended to regard the commission as long overdue. Through their spokesmen a number of these hospitals made public statements expressing their approval of the commission's formation and mandate. The OHA's official position, however, as expressed by its president, was critical of the government's decision to put power over the future of hospitals in the hands of a small group of nonelected people. The OHA and the small hospitals that make up the majority of its dues-paying membership were suspicious about this new, untried decision-making process replacing familiar ones that permitted direct contact between each hospital and its MPP, with or without the OHA, and the minister/Ministry of Health. Unlike the leaders of the great majority of health care organizations — the OMA, the Catholic Health Association of Ontario, the Association of District Health Councils of Ontario and the like — the relatively new OHA president, David MacKinnon, did not meet with the chair of the commission until well into the fall of 1996, after the OHA's annual meeting.[20] At that meeting, Sinclair, speaking to a large audience, admitted, to the consternation of many hospital representatives in attendance, that the two men had never met. MacKinnon not only was opposed to the commission as an "off-line" maker of decisions that should have been made by government, but he also took exception to the chair's saying publicly that he had accepted the job in part because he considered it "his duty to his grandchildren." This inauspicious beginning of the relationship between Sinclair and MacKinnon affected relations between the commission and the OHA for the next four years.

The Catholic Health Association of Ontario and its membership of hospitals owned and governed by Catholic orders or their successor — that is, the Catholic Health Corporation of Ontario,[21] the umbrella group that has inherited ownership of those hospitals no longer owned by religious orders — was particularly nervous. It represented the smaller hospitals offering acute-care services in the majority of Ontario's two-hospital towns and cities. Although it felt especially threatened and met early on with the commission's chair and chief executive officer to emphasize the important contributions of faith-based institutions to hospital care in Ontario, its public reaction was restrained.

Although there was some media interest in the commission's formation, in particular on the part of the print media, subsequent to passage of the enabling legislation published commentary was sporadic and relatively favourable, at least until the initial reports on hospital restructuring began to appear in the fall of 1996. An ominous commentary appeared in *The Globe and Mail* early on under the headline "Travelling Executioners to Seal Fate of Ontario Hospitals": "For Ontario hospitals, the Grim Reaper has assumed a new form. Over the next 18 months, the province's Health Services Restructuring Commission will be travelling across Ontario deciding which hospitals will live and which will die" (Rusk 1996).

When the HSRC was "in town" subsequently, local media coverage of its activities and announced intentions was intense. Although some media reacted negatively to the commission's initial reports in the communities studied first, Thunder Bay and Pembroke, even there the coverage of the commission's work, decisions and recommendations was balanced and, on the whole, favourable. The commissioners and their staff had anticipated very negative treatment of their decisions by media in the communities affected. They were pleasantly surprised by the balanced reporting and editorial commentary published in most communities subsequent to the commission's release of its reports.

Among the general public there was little reaction to the commission's formation. Public interest was piqued subsequently by the commission's initial proposals (called *Notices*) and final decisions (called *Directions*), community by community, but it was largely confined to supporters of the hospitals affected.

This muted and generally supportive reaction came as somewhat of a surprise to the commission, which had anticipated much more vigorous and vociferous opposition to its very formation, all played out in the spotlight of negative media coverage. It was taken as a sign that perhaps the people of Ontario accepted the need for change in health care, even when it affected acute-care hospitals, the system's most visible (and expensive) icons. As time passed and the HSRC worked through its mandate, the commissioners became more and more impressed with the perceived willingness of the general public to entertain discussion about radical changes in the organization and delivery of health services in Ontario. The members of the public with whom the commission interacted seemed far more willing than the government or hospitals, physicians, nurses and other health care providers to contemplate anything but the most modest changes to the status quo. Dr. Arnold Aberman, a former dean of medicine at the University of Toronto, addressing an audience of physicians, summed up the situation with a joke. "Question: How many doctors does it take to change a light bulb? Answer: Change?"

Appendix 1
SOME ELEMENTS OF BILL 26

The *Savings and Restructuring Act* contained the framework for the HSRC. Schedules F, G, H and I were the health package of the omnibus bill, which amended the *Ministry of Health Act*, the *Public Hospitals Act*, the *Private Hospitals Act* and the *Independent Health Facilities Act*.

Specifically pertaining to the Health Services Restructuring Commission was part 1 of schedule F of Bill 26:
- 1.8.(1) The Lieutenant Governor in Council may establish a body to be known in English as the Health Services Restructuring Commission.
- 1.8.(2) The members of the commission shall be appointed by the Lieutenant Governor in Council.
- 1.8.(3) The commission shall be a corporation without share capital composed of the members of the commission from time to time.
- 1.8.(4) The *Corporations Act* does not apply to the commission, except as provided by the regulations.
- 1.8.(5) The *Corporations Information Act* does not apply to the commission.
- 1.8.(9) No proceeding for damages or otherwise shall be commenced against the commission or against a member, officer, employee or agent of the commission for any act done in good faith in the execution or intended execution of any of its or their powers or duties or for any alleged neglect or default in the execution in good faith of any of its or their powers or duties.

NOTES

1. Later merged with the Toronto General Hospital and still later with the Princess Margaret Hospital to form the University Health Network.
2. The Premier's Council on Health Strategy (Peterson) and the Premier's Council on Health, Well-Being and Social Justice (Rae).
3. The model proposed in the Orser report was quite complex. While the regional board would have responsibility for overseeing the system, under it would be six Area Health Management Boards and a Regional Health Sciences Management Board. The area boards would have responsibilities similar to those of DHCs; area residents were to be appointed as their members.
4. Charles Bigenwald, Executive Director, Hospitals Branch, Ontario Ministry of Health, personal communication to HSRC, 1996.
5. For example, the partnership between the Sault Ste. Marie General and the Plummer Memorial, and the merger of the Toronto Western and the Toronto General (now the University Health Network).
6. The Windsor and Toronto DHCs are good examples.
7. Subsequently rescinded.
8. Ontario's *Public Hospitals Act* was first proclaimed in 1931. Since that time, the Act and its regulations have been further developed and revised to accommodate changing circumstances.
9. See appendix 1 for details of the regulations.
10. Schedule F amended the *Ministry of Health Act*, the *Public Hospitals Act*, the *Private Hospitals Act* and the *Independent Health Facilities Act*. Schedule G amended the *Ontario Drug Benefit Act*, the *Prescription Drug Cost Regulation Act* and the *Regulated Health Professions Act, 1991*. Schedule H amended the *Health Insurance Act* and the *Health Care Accessibility Act*. Schedule I amended the *Physician Services Delivery Management Act, 1995*.
11. O. Reg. 87/96 and 88/96.
12. Regulations under the *Ministry of Health Act* and the *Public Hospitals Act* gave the commission its powers and duties. These regulations were filed on March 22, 1996, as O. Reg. 87/96 (under the *Public Health Act*) and O. Reg. 88/96 (under the *Ministry of Health Act*) and came into force on April 1, 1996. The powers given to the commission in these two regulations, together with the provisions in section 8 of the *Ministry of Health Act* and sections 6 and 9(10) of the *Public Hospitals Act*, comprised all of the powers and authority of the commission.
13. In 1988 Congress enacted *Public Law 100-526*, creating the Secretary of Defense's Commission on Base Realignment and Closure (BRAC) and giving it the authority to recommend installations for closure or realignment based on an independent study of the domestic military base structure. In 1988 the commission recommended the closure of 86 installations and the realignment of 59. BRAC was estimated to generate savings of $693.6 million annually. The declining force structure of the post-Cold War era brought the need for additional closures and realignments, but by then the commission's charter had expired. In 1990, under the guidance of Secretary Cheney, the Executive Branch announced additional closures and realignments, but Congress rejected the proposal. To break the impasse, Congress created an independent five-year Defense Base Closure and Realignment Commission. The new law required the commission to hold public hearings on the secretary of defense's closure list, and the records were open to the public. The commission independently reviewed the secretary's recommendations and submitted its findings to the president. The General Accounting Office was required to review the report, provide a detailed analysis of the secretary's recommendations and submit its findings to the commission.
14. To date, Ontario, Nunavut and Yukon have not regionalized the delivery of health services.

15 Depending on the province, some members are elected locally.
16 In Saskatchewan, 435 such boards were replaced by 30 district boards. In the past two years there has also been a pattern of collapsing the number of RHAs in most jurisdictions.
17 Clair (Quebec), Fyke (Saskatchewan) and Mazankowski (Alberta).
18 The steering committee was established to carry out a comprehensive review of the Act and advise the minister of health on changes that would enable public hospitals to respond effectively to current and future health care needs in Ontario.
19 Now the Department of Health Policy, Management and Evaluation.
20 MacKinnon and Mark Rochon, chief executive officer of the commission, did meet in the summer of 1996.
21 Incorporated under civil and canon law, the CHCO is a partnership of the Catholic Health Association of Ontario and four religious congregations (the Grey Sisters of the Immaculate Conception, Pembroke; the Sisters of St. Joseph, Toronto; the Sisters of St. Joseph, Sault Ste. Marie; and the Sisters of Charity, Ottawa). Its main role is to ensure a Catholic presence in the health care institutions it sponsors. The institutions continue to operate as separate corporations in a manner consistent with the teachings of the Catholic Church, as well as complying with the *Health Care Ethics Guide*, published by the Catholic Health Association of Canada.

CHAPTER 2

THE POLICY CONTEXT

The health-policy environment in Ontario in the mid-1990s was dominated, as it has been throughout Canada since that time, by growing unease, tending to concern and even alarm that Medicare, that most cherished of social programs, was in trouble. The newspapers were full of stories about lengthening waiting lists for diagnostic services, access to hospital beds and specialist services, and increasing difficulty in securing a family physician, especially in small and medium-sized communities and in the North. A growing segment of the population was beginning to doubt that health care would be "there" for them when they and their children needed it.

Well aware of the effect of Canada's high tax rates on Canada's global competitiveness, governments and taxpayers alike were deeply worried about health care's appetite for annual increases in funding over and above both the general rate of inflation and the growth of government tax revenues. As a one-time minister of finance in Saskatchewan has recently written (MacKinnon 2004), Canada's spending on health care is among the highest in the world. It was 7 percent of GDP in 1975, but when the data are in for the year 2003 it is likely to have reached 10 percent — and this is an underestimate of the total, given that it excludes the accumulated debts of hospitals and health authorities and the capital cost of replacing fully depreciated buildings and equipment; in Ontario alone this is estimated to exceed $100 billion. The Conference Board of Canada (McIntyre, O'Sullivan and Frank 2003) has pointed out that spending on health care not only claims the lion's share of total provincial/territorial expenditures, but that this share is increasing at an alarming rate, growing from 32 percent in 2001 to 38 percent in 2003; it is forecast to consume an average of 44 percent

(50 percent in Ontario and British Columbia[1]) by 2020. In Ontario, in the five-year period 1997-98 to 2002-03 health care spending increased by 42 percent; in the same period provincial revenues grew by 31 percent.

Signs of the subsequent upturn in the economy were still tentative in 1996. It is fair to say that the driving force behind the development and implementation of every health-related policy by Ontario's newly elected Progressive Conservative government was the need to contain costs and eliminate the deficit inherited from previous regimes. Funding and spending considerations dominated all health-policy discussions.

The concern over the fact that increases in the cost of health care continue to outstrip the rate of revenue increase of any government in Canada (except debt-free Alberta) remains coupled, eight years later, with increasingly bitter public wrangling over how those costs should be shared between the federal government, with its superior taxing authority, and the provinces and territories, with their primary responsibility for the provision of health care to Canadians.

In 1957, as an incentive to all provinces to develop publicly funded hospital insurance programs, the federal government offered to share the cost on a 50:50 basis; this was extended to publicly insured physician services in 1966. In 1977-78 this open-ended sharing arrangement was replaced by a block-funding transfer mechanism (Established Programs Financing, or EPF) in which each province received an equal per-capita transfer of a mixture of "tax points" and cash to support health care and postsecondary education together. Health care was said to constitute about 70 percent of the total, but the breakdown was entirely notional because EPF transfers were not linked to actual provincial expenditures on either health care or postsecondary education. Initially the cash transfer was subject to an escalator based on the observed growth in GDP per capita, but, to save money, between 1986-87 and 1995-96 the federal government adjusted the escalator downward several times. In 1995-96 Ottawa replaced EPF with a larger block-funding mechanism, the Canada Health and Social Transfer (CHST), to cover tax and cash transfers to the provinces and territories for social assistance as well as health care and postsecondary education. The CHST legislation, which was subsequently amended several times in quick succession, contained a cash floor to ensure that growth in the value of the transferred tax points would not erode the cash transfer to zero and thereby remove the power of the federal government to enforce the *Canada Health Act*.

The complexities of these block-transfer arrangements, their frequent amendment, and the lumping together of the three costly social programs administered by the provinces and territories, coupled with the earlier downward adjustments of the cash component of EPF financing, laid the ground for the current provincial/territorial case that Ottawa's contribution to the cost of health care in Canada has shrunk to as little as 16 percent of the total. Although the real share, taking both tax points and cash transfers into account, remains in dispute and the subject of repeated arcane accounting exercises, the most recent election campaign featured promises by all prime ministerial candidates to "put more money into health care." A consensus seems to be emerging that federal cash transfers to the provinces/territories approximating 25 percent of the total cost of publicly insured health services would be about right; sharp divisions remain, however, as to accountability — the strings that might be attached to such transfers. Apart from alleviating some provincial/territorial financial pressures, achieving the 25 percent target, with or without strings, might have a far more lasting effect. With squabbling over shared funding behind them, both levels of government might turn their focus to a more vital and productive issue — how to use the many policy changes that are needed in health care to create a genuine and sustainable health care system that meets the needs of Canadians and optimizes the health of the population into a future much different from that of the late 1950s and the 1960s, when Medicare was instituted.

When the Health Services Restructuring Commission came on the scene in 1996, getting more funds from the federal government was of particular concern to the Ontario government. In addition to diminishing health care's drain on the provincial treasury, funding decisions were, apart from exhortation, the principal if not the only tool the government had to steer hospitals, doctors and other providers toward its objectives for the system. Without money to spend, the health system's rudder did not work. Yet in those years the annual discussions between the premiers and the prime minister were no more fruitful (from a provincial perspective) than they had been in the preceding few years. Ottawa continued to give priority to eliminating its long-standing deficit, balancing its books and reducing the national debt — in large part by decreasing its spending, including that on transfer payments. It was an anxious and stressful time for everybody, not least the "have" province of Ontario, with its keen interest in policy decisions regarding equalization and related federal transfers to the "have not" provinces.

But the new government's long-term policy objectives for health care were no more explicit than those of its predecessors. The Tories in Ontario were no more eager than the New Democrats and Liberals before them to come to grips with the challenges of creating a real health care system — to provide it with leadership and direction by developing clear policies, goals and objectives by setting priorities and establishing the values it should adhere to in the process. To be fair, to put in place the processes and tools necessary to provide the health care system with effective governance and accountability where little or none had existed before would have been a Herculean challenge for any new government, much less one faced with enormous and acute fiscal problems. But it remains that when the commission began its work in the late spring of 1996 no effective governance — no real leadership — of health care as a putative system existed in Ontario, even though its components consumed huge amounts of public money and notwithstanding its all-too-obvious political and practical importance to the citizenry.

Of the policy initiatives, perhaps the freshest was the legacy of Premier David Peterson's Council on Health Strategy (1986-90) and Premier Bob Rae's Council on Health, Well-Being and Social Justice (1991-95). Both of these councils and their widely reported findings had built on and extended the currency of the landmark Lalonde report some years before, citing education, social security, housing and many other factors — in addition to health care services — as powerful determinants of health.[2] Among the many studies they conducted, the two consecutive premier's councils provided up-to-date, compelling evidence to make people aware of the relative importance of the many determinants of health that fall within the purview of government policy. They pointed out the opportunity cost to the health of the population over the long term of continued disproportionate spending on health. The same messages were being reinforced in the well-publicized work and final report of the Prime Minister's National Forum on Health (1994-97), released a year after the commission began its work (Prime Minister's National Forum on Health 1997). The opportunity-cost factor was very much on the minds of the commissioners. It stiffened their resolve to focus first on using the HSRC's unprecedented power to reorganize Ontario hospitals into the most efficient and cost-effective configuration possible and next on developing policies and strategies the government could use to integrate the work of hospitals with that of the many other service providers needed in a genuine system of health care.

Given the large number of apparently redundant beds in the system, the immediate policy objective of the government and the commission was to reduce the number of hospitals in the province — especially acute-care hospitals — without diminishing either the accessibility or the quality of their services. This objective was coupled, at least by the commission, with that of ensuring the availability of alternative, community-based services in sufficient quantity and quality to meet the needs of patients who did not require hospitalization but were not well enough to be sent home without care. The primary goal, in addition to achieving greater cost-effectiveness, was to demonstrate dramatically the need for a change in health care and the fact that this could be achieved even in institutions as precious as hospitals. Just as important was the need to shift capacity and resources from hospital-based to equally effective but less expensive forms of care, particularly home care and long-term care.

The new government's commitment to these goals can be inferred from two policy decisions made shortly after the Conservatives were elected in 1995 — that the funding envelope for hospitals be reduced by 18 percent over the next three fiscal years, and that the budget of the Ministry of Health, also the main source of funding for other publicly funded providers of health services, not be reduced throughout their term in office. After the many years when hospitals consistently claimed funding priority over virtually all other providers, the shift away from hospital care as a priority was dramatic. This shift was strongly reinforced, of course, by the introduction of and debate over the legislation creating the HSRC, showing very clearly that the new government was serious about making a change and making it quickly — serious enough to take politics out of the equation by handing the task (and the necessary power) over to an independent third party. Nevertheless, in announcing its decision to protect the total budget of the Ministry of Health when virtually everything else was subject to substantial and repeated cuts, the government also made it clear that, from a policy perspective, health care was at the top of its priority list and would continue to claim that position throughout its term in office.

Reassuring as this policy pronouncement was intended to be, it gained little or no credit within the health care system, where expectations ran high for salary and wage increases. Throughout Ontario at the time, the mood of public and quasi-public servants was particularly truculent following the imposition, by the previous government, of "Rae Days" — days off without pay to reduce the salary and wage burden. The result of the failure to negotiate a "social contract," Rae Days were intended to avert a fiscal crisis in the early 1990s brought on by a combination of the economic downturn and the disastrous decision by the

NDP government soon after its election to spend its way out of the recession. This initiative had the effect of reducing government spending, including spending on those organizations that were primarily government-funded. Not surprisingly, the fact that the new Conservative government's prioritization of health care did not extend to raising substantially salaries and wages was regarded, by physicians, hospitals, other health care organizations and health care workers, as not giving them much priority at all. High expectations added to the government's preoccupation with money and where and how to find more of it.

THE NEED FOR POLICY

Despite the predominance of financial considerations in Ontario in the mid-1990s, throughout Canada the many issues crying out for the development of forward-looking health policy kept health ministers and their more thoughtful senior bureaucrats awake at night. None of the issues were new then and all have continued to grow more serious in terms of their claim on public attention. The obvious ones have been described succinctly and well by the Standing Senate Committee on Social Affairs, Science and Technology (2002a). They include:
> aging of the population and its potential effects on the provision and financing of health care
> increasing demand for and cost of new diagnostic and therapeutic technologies, including drugs
> health human resource issues, especially shortages of physicians and other health professionals in remote, rural and small communities
> inadequacies of health information management
> meeting the particular health needs of Aboriginal populations
> disease trends: the re-emergence of "old" diseases and the appearance of new ones
> rebalancing approaches to preventive measures affecting health in the long term with the short-term imperatives of providing sickness care

To this list the commission would have added:
> mental health services, especially those available to people who remain in their communities
> home care

Canada's aging population is said to be "one of the great successes of the health and social services systems."[3] Although there is room for argument about the causative effects of those systems versus other factors, the proportion of Canadians 65 and over rose from 4.1 to 9.7 percent of the population in the century ending in 1981; while seniors constituted 12.5 percent of all Canadians in 2000, they are projected to constitute a quarter of the population 50 years hence. And, happily for those of us who are seniors now, the old are getting older: by 2051, when the last of the baby boomers turns 85, the proportion of the cohort that age and over is expected to reach 21 percent of all seniors. The bad news is that the cost of providing seniors with health services (as they are provided now) increases exponentially, doubling from age 45-64 by decade through age 65-74, 75-84 to 85 and over. This has led to the development of the "nightmare high cost," "compressed morbidity," "manageable costs" and "reformed system" models,[4] four scenarios to use as starting points for developing policies to optimize the health of this expanding segment of the population without bankrupting the reduced number of working-age Canadian taxpayers. It is a daunting but not impossible task. The Senate committee observed that "the United States spends close to 14% of its GDP on health care but the proportion of seniors in its population is less than 13%, whereas Sweden spends less than 9%... even though its proportion of seniors is 17%...and their life expectancy is higher."[5] But the task is impossible without a fundamental change in the way health services have been provided since the introduction of medicare.

When the commission began its work in 1996, just as the high expectations of health care and other workers in the public and quasi-public sectors created a particular challenge in the policy environment, so too did the expectations of all Canadians for greater access to new diagnostic and therapeutic technologies — imaging machines like CTs and MRIs,[6] radiation therapy, coronary artery stents, replacement hips, knees and lenses, and an ever-increasing array of prescription drugs. Such changing public expectations relating to quick and easy access to high-quality services constitute one of the four "winds"[7] affecting contemporary health care that remain to be fully accommodated in the policy framework that supports its provision everywhere (Decter 2000). To illustrate, on one of his weekly train commutes from his home in Kingston, the commission's chair chanced to sit beside a woman from Boston, a Canadian-born and -educated clinical psychologist returning to Toronto for the first time in many years. On discovering his involvement in health care, she averred that she would not be comfortable living in Canada now due to her concern about access to health care here. She said it was her understanding that there were more MRI machines in the city of Boston than in all of Ontario, perhaps even all of Canada. The legions of Americans without health insurance and the extraordinary leap of logic necessary to connect MRI scans with good health did not enter the picture. Given Canada's propinquity to the United States and its advertising of such imaging, drugs, eye surgery and all manner of health services as commodities, it would be surprising were the northern wind of public expectation not blowing ever more strongly based more on the desire for quick gratification of induced demand than on genuine medical necessity.

Canadian Medicare is founded on the principle that access to hospital and physician care should be based on need and not, as with commercial goods and services, on ability to pay. Logically, waiting lists should also differentiate between need and demand, with those in greatest need at the top. Yet in the mid-1990s, when the commission began its work and long waits for access to many health services, including new technologies, was widely acknowledged to be a serious problem, Ontario had only one real waiting list, that of the Cardiac Care Network. It was the sole disciplined list functioning on the basis of criteria to determine, province-wide, patients' relative need for cardiac surgery and, later, angiography. Although progress has since been made — by, for example, Cancer Care Ontario for some cancer services and, in Saskatchewan and Alberta, for surgical and some other services — the great majority of the waiting lists that are causing angst among the public and hand-wringing by providers and health ministers alike are still maintained by individual physicians and/or institutions and are based on idiosyncratic criteria that may or may not differentiate between need and demand. A formidable policy challenge is how to reach consensus, among providers and consumers, on appropriate criteria and their application to genuine, fair waiting lists that will support credible measurement of patients' relative need (as opposed to demand) for the expensive new technologies, including pharmaceutical agents, that continue to be introduced into health care.

In the absence of such policies and appropriately ordered waiting lists, the best Canada and its provinces and territories can do is to compare themselves with other countries and jurisdictions. On that score it does appear that Canadians everywhere have less access to new technologies, especially diagnostic equipment like MRIs, than they should.

Spending on drugs has increased dramatically. From a relatively steady base of between 8 and 9 percent of total health expenditures in the period 1975-84, spending on drugs has grown, exceeding the rate of inflation, in an almost linear fashion, to 16 percent in 2003 (Canadian Institute for Health Information [CIHI] and Statistics Canada 2004); since 1997 it has exceeded the total spent in every category but hospital care. The federal Patent Medicine Prices Review Board limits annual increases in the price of patented drugs to increases in the Consumer Price Index. In addition, provinces and territories use generic substitution, formulary management, reference-based pricing and other methods to control the rate of cost increases. One of the main cost drivers (thought to explain about 30 percent of the rate of increase) is the greater use each year of new, more costly drugs. Another cost driver is utilization; Health Canada reports that 8.9 prescriptions were dispensed per person in 1999, an increase of 6.3 percent over 1998 (Standing Senate Committee 2002a, 22). Among the economic costs of drug therapy are inappropriate prescribing by physicians (of antibiotics for colds and other viral infections, for example) and inappropriate and inconsistent use by patients — failure to comply with the instructions of the physician and/or pharmacist. For some years the provinces have wrestled with the twin measures of putting policies in place to control the rate of increase in spending on prescription drugs and finding affordable ways to remove ability to pay as a barrier to access to medical technologies. It remains, however, that access to drug therapies is at best "two tier" and more often "three tier" (publicly insured, privately insured and uninsured) throughout Canada.

HEALTH HUMAN RESOURCES

When the commission was established in 1996, health human resources, particularly perceived shortages of physicians and nurses, were very much on the minds of the provincial and territorial governments. Reviewing this issue in 2002, two years after the HSRC closed its doors, the Standing Senate Committee pointed out that whereas the workforce of registered (7 percent) and licensed (17 percent) practical nurses per 100,000 Canadians had decreased significantly in the 1990s, the comparable population of physicians had hardly changed (0.5 percent) while those of most other health professionals — pharmacists, dentists, physiotherapists and so on — had increased, some substantially (e.g., dental hygienists by 59 percent [2002a]). In Ontario, according to figures maintained by the Ontario Physician Human Resources Data Centre, the supply of physicians relative to population has declined steadily, from 186 per 100,000 people in 1995 to 175 in 2000 (Ontario Medical Association Human Resources Committee 2002); the most recent data show a net loss of 110 active physicians between 1999 and 2000, and dramatic year-over-year decreases in some specialties. In 1999 an independent fact-finder concluded that Ontario had a shortage of about 1,000 physicians and that a 5 percent increase in overall physician supply was required (McKendry 1999). In 2001 the College of Family Physicians of Canada estimated that Ontario required a minimum increase of 1,000 family physicians. A 2002 report from the Institute for Clinical Evaluative Sciences shows that the physician supply in Ontario peaked in 1993 and has since dropped by 5 percent, to the 1987 level (Chan 2002); the supply estimates account for population aging, more intense use of health services by the elderly and the fact that a growing number of physicians are women, who, on average, work fewer hours than their male colleagues. As with all workforces, the consideration of shortages and surpluses of health professionals must include, in addition to the number available, their productivity, distribution throughout the jurisdiction and the extent to which their services could be provided by others.

Nursing in its various forms constitutes some two-thirds of the health care workforce in Canada. Traditionally a profession populated by women, worldwide it has not fared well in competition with the ever-widening array of other careers that have become open to women over the last few decades. The number of new Canadian graduates in nursing dropped from about 10,000 per year in the 1970s to 8,000 in the 1980s and 5,500 in 1995. In 1997 the Canadian Nurses Association forecast a shortfall of nearly 60,000 registered nurses by 2011, and as many as 113,000 if the needs of the aging population for nursing care are taken fully into account (Ryten 1997). Compounding factors are the instability of employment faced by hospital-based nurses (the high proportion of part-time nurses constitutes hospitals' buffer against financial shortfalls) and higher pay and better working conditions in the United States. With the HSRC's initial focus on rationalizing Ontario's urban hospitals, there was some fear that even more nurses would be laid off and out of work. However, the prime policy consideration at the time was ways and means of recruiting more young people to the profession and retaining experienced nurses frustrated by the insecurity of their increasingly casual/part-time status in hospitals, stressful working conditions and lack of respect and status, especially relative to physicians. Compounding the issue were policy decisions, driven primarily by the profession itself, to restrict RN status to those who had completed a four-year baccalaureate closing the previous route of entry provided by Ontario's community colleges. Despite long-standing recognition of the magnitude and seriousness of the shortage of qualified nursing personnel and the impending crisis as experienced nurses continue to leave the profession through retirement, recruitment to positions in the United States, or the pursuit of less stressful and more satisfying careers, nobody seems to be working very hard on developing and implementing long-range policy solutions.

Although shortages of doctors, especially family physicians offering comprehensive primary care, are obvious, their causes and potential remedies are both unclear and in dispute. Whereas increases in the number of specialists in Canada outpaced population growth between 1995 and 2000, the supply of family physicians did drop slightly, from 95 to 94 per 100,000 people (CIHI 2001), hardly sufficient to explain the decreasing availability of primary care, which is especially marked outside Canada's major cities. Much has been made of decisions by provincial governments to order a 10 percent decrease in medical school enrolments following the release of a 1991 report identifying physicians as Medicare's dominant cost-generators; the recommended decrease in intake at the undergraduate level was coupled with others related to the training of graduates of foreign medical schools, financing academic medical centres, postgraduate (residency) training, and other changes to improve the productivity of education and, subsequently, of the system (Barer and Stoddart 1991). Sadly the report was not adopted as a whole; the policy of reduced undergraduate medical education was "cherry-picked," mainly because it was easier to implement than the companion recommendations. In any case, given the long duration of medical education and training, the impact of reduced undergraduate enrolment did not begin to come online until 1998-99; it certainly neither caused nor contributed to the shortage of family physicians in remote, rural and small-town Ontario and throughout Canada in the 1990s and earlier. The apparent shortage can be attributed to a number of factors:

> the decrease in the number of practising family and general physicians
> the failure of newly qualified physicians to take over the rural and small-town practices of aging doctors, who reduce their workloads for a while and then retire
> the choice of newly qualified physicians to practise in cities close to specialists and teaching hospitals and other institutions to which their more complicated and time-consuming cases can be referred

> the increase in the number of family physicians who no longer provide comprehensive primary care (including obstetrics) but restrict their practices to patients with a narrow range of health problems — counselling, sports medicine, podiatry and so forth
> lifestyle choices, particularly on the part of the increasing proportion of women in medicine, in favour of group practice, a shorter work week, little or no on-call duty, and more opportunity to balance the demands of professional and family life
> the greater opportunities offered in big cities to two-career families

In Ontario, the decrease in undergraduate enrolment was coupled with the government's introduction of strict caps on the total number of postgraduate or residency positions, equivalent to the number of graduates, and on their distribution among family medicine and the various specialties. This precluded continuation of a long-standing model whereby physicians in large numbers would, after a few years in family practice, re-enter postgraduate training, typically in anesthesiology, emergency medicine, general medicine, surgery or pathology, and return, after qualifying, to provide specialty services in their local community hospital. It also had the disadvantage of encouraging undergraduates to choose a residency program at an early stage in their education before they had sufficient experience to know what they were getting into (and it was difficult to switch programs later). The universities were also allowed to raise tuition in medicine and other professional programs to compensate for increases in government grants that failed to match the rate of inflation (another opportunity cost); the debt loads of medical students grew and, naturally, in their choice of residency they continued to be tempted by the higher-earning specialties — rejecting family medicine and the generalist specialties most needed in small communities. The opportunities for foreign-trained physicians to qualify for licensure to practice in Ontario were also tightly controlled by exceedingly parsimonious rationing of earmarked residency positions. All of these health human resource policies, intended to limit physician-induced cost pressures on the system, continued for about a decade, until the policy on undergraduate admissions was abruptly reversed, enrolments in medical schools were greatly expanded and a new, sixth, medical school, slated to accept its first students in 2005, was established in northern Ontario. Will this sort of crude "supply management" of health human resources correct maldistribution and the doctor shortage? Not likely.

HEALTH INFORMATION MANAGEMENT

Perhaps the most consequential of the policy vacuums the commission encountered in 1996 was that related to health information — its standardization (or lack thereof), recording, transmission, sharing, storage, analysis, utilization both clinically and for management and accountability purposes, security, and the rules necessary to balance its effective use against the privacy rights of the individuals concerned, both patients and providers. At the foundation of health information are electronic and other health records that fully inform doctors and others regarding a person's health status and history of interactions with care providers. Included in the concept of health information are networks to inform the public and help them make sense of the many thousands of Internet sites that purport to offer useful information on health and disease. Included also is the concept of telemedicine/telecare to enable timely, appropriate and beneficial interactions at a distance between patients and health care providers such as doctors, nurses, home-care case managers and counsellors — enhancing the *Canada Health Act*'s principle of accessibility, especially for people in remote and rural areas. Continuing education and training of health care providers at a distance also falls within the rubric of information and communication technology (ICT) or, more properly, management (ICM). For some time, frankly, the availability of sophisticated ICT has surpassed the ability to manage and use it well in health care, an information-intensive field if ever there was one. The cost and compatibility of ICT are indeed issues, but far more important are the policies and leadership necessary to optimize its effectiveness.

There are three barriers to the development, implementation and deployment of a comprehensive and effective health information and communication management system, provincially and, ultimately, nationally:

> lack of standardization to the extent necessary for information to be shared — so it will convey the same meaning to every person who has access to it, including the most important person of all, the patient who is its subject and owner

> legal and ethical challenges to the protection of personal information

> lack of interoperability of a wide variety of technologies and protocols

Surmounting these barriers will require strong leadership of many diverse and often divergent interests — leadership that the commission saw no evidence of in the Ontario government of the mid-1990s. There was no policy in place to provide for the development of standards whether applied to data or to communication among different computer-based systems. The health ministry was only one of several entities wrestling with draft privacy legislation to protect personal information in ways that would meet Ontario's needs from the perspective of all players and yet be consistent with draft legislation in Ottawa intended to set nationwide standards of privacy, confidentiality and security.[8] The ministry's ICT initiative, Smart Systems for Health, working on the interoperability of technologies and protocols, among other things, and in place before the commission was formed, has proved unsuccessful as a consolidating force among the many institutional and individual participants in the health care system. Much of the estimated $500 million that was spent annually in Ontario on ICT/M will prove to have been wasted for want of strong policy leadership on the part of the government as a whole. The ministry's declaration of e-health as a priority may represent a more recent ray of hope.

ABORIGINAL AND POPULATION HEALTH

Although the provision of health services to Aboriginal populations is a federal responsibility, the notoriously poor health of Aboriginal people, off- as well as on-reserve, demands the attention of four levels of government: federal, provincial, municipal and Aboriginal. Aboriginal health constitutes a vivid example of how interplay among the determinants of health — housing, education, community services, employment, income security, wealth, self-actualization, genetics, and the social and physical environment, as well as preventive and therapeutic care — affects individuals and populations alike, both in the short and the long term. Despite the attention directed, over many years, to ways and means of improving Aboriginal health, and the dozens if not hundreds of reports written, studied and shelved, there is still no coordinated platform of policies to address the fact that this population experiences poorer health, shorter life expectancy, higher infant mortality and higher rates of a variety of chronic illnesses than Canadians as a whole.[9] It is a significant policy issue that remains to be addressed throughout Canada.

Changes in the pattern of diseases away from infectious diseases and toward noncommunicable, chronic diseases can be credited to improvements in the efficacy of health care — as well as to education, access to clean water, proper nutrition and so on — throughout the twentieth century. Cardiovascular disease, cancer and accidents are now the three leading causes of death in Canada. Not all infectious diseases have been conquered, however; the provision of care for patients with antibiotic-resistant tuberculosis was an issue the HSRC had to consider when restructuring Ontario's public hospitals. The outbreak of SARS in Toronto and elsewhere illustrates the danger of complacency about the threat of new infectious diseases, especially given the swift, modern transport of people, animals and foodstuffs throughout the world (Expert Panel on SARS and Infectious Disease Control 2004).

SARS also illustrates the folly of concentrating a large proportion of resources in the infrastructure and maintenance of sickness care at the expense of vigilance, readiness and effectiveness in preventive, public and population health — another of many opportunity costs. One extraordinarily misguided policy decision made by the newly elected Conservative government in 1995 was to shift total responsibility for the funding of Ontario's public health units to the already overstretched property-tax base of municipalities. Happily, this decision was partially and, after SARS, fully reversed. It illustrates, however, the relatively feeble claim at the time of preventive, public and population health on the attention of policy-makers. It also illustrates the government's preoccupation with financial issues; the shift of public health costs to municipalities was made in large part to "balance" the province's assumption of full responsibility for funding elementary and secondary education; it was an accounting exercise to benefit the provincial "books."

With respect to population-health strategies, there remain real obstacles, practical and political, to their application in the form of programs that are sustainable over the long haul. ParticipAction, the federal government's advertising campaign to encourage Canada's couch potatoes to exercise, is a case in point. Given the many factors that influence health outcomes, it is difficult to link definitively interventions promoting healthy populations with their outcomes, especially when the latter are realized only cumulatively and measured many years later, well beyond usual political horizons. Nevertheless, few would dispute the need for every society to put in place a robust policy framework around preventive, public and population health strategies and to provide the resources necessary to implement them. These matters were not high on the policy agenda of the Ministry of Health, or the government more broadly, when the commission began its work in 1996. Because of SARS, they have higher priority now.

MENTAL HEALTH

Mention must be made of mental health policy in Ontario. Difficult to diagnose and define, mental illness has been estimated to affect 3 percent of Canadians of all ages in ways that significantly impair their work, social interactions and ability to function independently in their communities.[10] Like most provinces, for many years Ontario governed and administered directly, through the Ministry of Health, a number of Provincial Psychiatric Hospitals (PPHs) that provided both in-patient and outpatient care for people with mental disorders, primarily those of a chronic, long-term nature. Acute mental health services were provided primarily in and by the same general hospitals that provided an array of other hospital-based services, although the distinctions between what those public hospitals and PPHs did were far from clear. Following a policy decision taken abruptly in the 1970s, many long-stay patients were discharged from PPHs without adequate arrangements being made to prepare them or the recipient communities for the change in their accommodation and care. Subsequently, it is fair to say, policy considerations relating to the care, treatment and accommodation of people with mental disorders remained a high priority, at least for study by the Ministry of Health; a number of insightful reports[11] were available to the commission when it began its work, although little action had been taken on their recommendations. Among the many issues involved was the stigma of mental illness, created in part by the fact that mental health services were to a great extent "hived off," including in PPHs, from the services and institutions available for the care of people with illnesses affecting other bodily systems. A fundamental policy decision had to be made whether to integrate all health services or continue with separate ones for mental health.

HOME CARE

Another policy issue very much "in play" relates to home care, a mixture of social-support services to help aging people remain longer in their residential settings with the professional caregiving that is characteristic of health services. Aging of the population and diminished availability of hospital beds, coupled with the availability of new knowledge and technology facilitating the safe provision of interventions out of hospital by nurses and others rather than by physicians, resulted in rapid expansion of the use of home-care services during the 1980s and 1990s. Health Canada reported a pattern of accelerated growth in public spending on home care, from well under $100 million in 1975-76 to over $2 billion annually in 1997-98, increasing in the 1990s by 11 percent a year (2001). Data on the out-of-pocket costs of home care borne by clients and their families are not readily available, but these costs have been estimated to cover approximately 60 percent of the bill for home-support services, 25 percent of the bill for nursing services and a smaller percentage of the bill for drugs, which, when prescribed out of hospital, are not covered under Medicare but are partially covered by publicly funded programs in most provinces. In 1999 the *Globe and Mail* estimated that home-care clients paid approximately $800 for nursing services, $410 for home support and $140 for prescription drugs, a total of $1,350 per month — an amount beyond the means of people in the low-income brackets, who, experience shows, have the greatest need for such services (Picard 1999). From a societal perspective, however, the vast majority of clients can be cared for at home at much less cost than in an acute-care or continuing-care hospital and, importantly, home care is strongly preferred by the recipients and their families.

Until the mid-1990s in Ontario, home-care services were provided by provincially funded regional agencies both directly by their employees and under contract with private organizations offering care on a not-for-profit and for-profit basis. Client access to care was in accordance with criteria set by the Ministry of Health and administered by case managers in the home-care agencies. These agencies were succeeded by Community Care Access Centres (CCACs) under the direction of local boards whose members (and chief executive officers) are appointed by the province. CCACs manage client access to home and long-term care and supervise the services provided to clients exclusively under contracts tendered to and negotiated with not-for-profit and for-profit private agencies. Initially CCACs operated within the limits of annual budgetary envelopes and with a small degree of independence; currently, however, to all intents and purposes they are arms of the ministry. The policy framework to provide greater continuity of care for patients who, subsequent to hospitalization, require home care and long-term care, however, remains to be developed to the point where it can be formalized in appropriate legislation.

DEVOLUTION

All of these issues were very much in play, not only in Ontario but in every province, when the commission was established in 1996. Where Ontario differed most was with respect to its centralized approach to micromanagement, by regulation and through its funding lever, of the many elements constituting the so-called health care system. Although the province began to experiment with devolution in 1974 by establishing District Health Councils made up of respected members of the communities concerned, staffing them to perform planning functions, the DHCs were never given any real authority. Many DHCs did excellent work — the reviews a number of them conducted of hospital-based services in their districts were invaluable to the commission in its hospital-restructuring phase — but their boards and staff members grew dispirited when much of their advice was not acted upon and their mandates seemed to be shrinking rather than expanding. By the mid-1990s all other provinces had taken the decision to devolve to regional health boards/authorities some degree of responsibility for planning, managing and governing parts of the spectrum of health care providers in their regions. Regionalization extended even to Prince Edward Island, although that province's total population and land mass are smaller than those of provinces served by most if not all other health authorities. As one of the commissioners has said elsewhere:

> Like everything else, devolution has its strengths and weaknesses. Principal among its strengths are:
>
> > Devolution distinguishes between the roles of governance and management. It requires government to do for health care what it alone can do — govern the system — including the important function of evaluating the performance of the managers on the ground to whom responsibility and authority has been devolved.
>
> > Devolution shifts managerial decision-making closer to those most affected, a shift that creates a greater sense of ownership in those decisions, in their outcomes, and in the processes used to make them.
>
> > Decisions can be more closely tailored to meet identified local/regional needs. It can diminish the "one size fits all" problem.

> Devolution establishes two-way accountability for how health services are delivered:
> - directly to representatives of the people affected and
> - to central governments, including for adherence to policies designed to preserve inter-regional and national equity.
> It fosters integration of services at a local (do-able) level.
> It offers the potential of depoliticizing many of the difficult prioritizing and rationing decisions that always have to be made in health care.

Devolution, of course, has its disadvantages too:
> It will add a layer of bureaucracy and additional administrative cost unless government ministries are "downsized" proportionate to the shift of management responsibilities. And bureaucracies don't shrink happily.
> Governments will fear loss of their illusory ability to co-ordinate the provision of services centrally.
> Sharing equitably sophisticated province- or nation-wide services located in one region with other regions can lead to very complex cost- and benefit-sharing calculations and procedures.
> The central bargaining power of a single large buyer of health care may be diminished.
> "Envelope" funding may offer the opportunity for governments to wriggle off the hook for adequate funding.
> Getting local/district/regional leaders to serve has been and may continue to be a problem.
> There are both up- and downsides to reduced political visibility for ministers and elected members of provincial/territorial legislatures.
> Two main opponents of devolution are hospital boards (who fear a loss of managerial control) and physicians (of central bargaining power). (Flood and Sinclair 2005)

Despite its resolute opposition to the policy of shifting power away from the centre, that is precisely what the Ontario government did by creating the Health Services Restructuring Commission, vesting in it the power of the government itself to restructure the province's public hospitals. Just why successive Ontario governments have been opposed to regionalization has never been fully explained, but it is clear that Ontario's policy of central command and control is increasingly at odds with the policies of all the other provinces.

INITIATIVES ELSEWHERE

Notwithstanding the continuing development of regional health boards/authorities as powerful forces in health care, throughout the 1990s every province was, to a greater or lesser degree, wrestling with the same policy issues as Ontario — and with the same small measure of success. Everywhere, spending on health care was growing faster than the rate of increase in government revenues, the opportunity costs to education and other publicly supported services were becoming obvious, the economy was not particularly robust (Alberta being an exception) and it was increasingly clear that some new thinking was required. Around the time that the HSRC reached its legislated "sunset" in 2000, similar bodies were established to provide that new thinking in three provinces. These were the Clair Commission (Commission d'étude sur les services de santé et les services sociaux) in Quebec, the Fyke Commission on Medicare in Saskatchewan and the Mazankowski Council in Alberta;[12] the mandate of the latter was to provide strategic advice to the Alberta premier on the preservation and enhancement of health services and on the continuing sustainability of Alberta's publicly funded and publicly administered health care system. Much shorter in duration than the HSRC, and lacking its power with regard to hospitals, these three advisory bodies nevertheless came to similar conclusions about the problems facing health care in their jurisdictions and what should be done about them.

Michel Clair (a former minister of Quebec's treasury board) and his colleagues pointed out, as the HSRC had done in its vision statement, that the problems facing health and social services were primarily organizational. Their resolution required a stark choice between the solidarity represented by Quebec's publicly funded health insurance program and an "every man for himself" philosophy — and the Clair Commission left no doubt that it stood on the side of the former. The Clair Commission stressed as a fundamental principle the obligation of all health care participants — governors, managers, health workers and recipients of care — to achieve the maximum benefits for the people of Quebec with the limited resources available for publicly funded services. Among its recommendations and proposals were topics very familiar to the members of the HSRC:

> disease prevention and health promotion should be the *central* element of Quebec's health and welfare policy
> secondary and tertiary care by hospitals and specialists should be consolidated into a hierarchical configuration to enhance accessibility to high-quality, cost-effective care
> networks of integrated services should be established, especially for the frail, elderly people with serious mental health problems and those with complex chronic diseases
> effective and secure clinical and management health information systems should be developed and implemented
> primary care should be reorganized; Family Medicine Groups (including nurse clinicians/practitioners) should provide health/medical care under a new, mixed or blended payment system, in collaboration with Centres local des services communautaires (CLSCs), long-established agencies unique to Quebec with responsibility for a range of health, psychosocial and community services
> the government should clearly define its role in governing Quebec's system of health and social services
> the government should devolve to regional boards responsibility for organizing services and allocating resources

Although very different from the Clair Commission and from one another in approach and style, the Fyke Commission and, later, the Mazankowski Council addressed the same themes in their in-depth analyses and policy recommendations:

> the need for change and leadership
> the need for a more systematic, integrated approach to providing the whole spectrum of essential services, from health promotion through tertiary and quaternary care
> the compelling need for a more hierarchical organization of hospitals, in accordance with the principle that those who do things frequently do them better and more cost-effectively

> the need to achieve greater quality and accountability through a vastly improved capacity for health information management based on electronic health records
> the need to replace the model of solo, fee-for-service family physicians with a system of multidisciplinary group practices offering an array of primary-care services 24 hours a day, 7 days a week

Looking back on the work of these four bodies focused on the challenge of providing health services in Ontario, Quebec, Saskatchewan and Alberta, one is struck by the consistency of their recommendations for changes in health policy. This consistency far outweighs their differences in relation to recommending ways and means of optimizing approaches to and implementation of those changes in the four very different jurisdictions.

Finally, this work in four provinces was complemented in 2002 by the release of two comprehensive reviews of health care in Canada, the six-volume report of the Standing Senate Committee, *The Health of Canadians: The Federal Role*, and the report of a Royal Commission, *Building on Values: The Future of Health Care in Canada*.

Reporting in November 2002, the sole member of the Royal Commission, Roy Romanow, a former premier of Saskatchewan, began his work in April 2001. He reviewed what had gone before — evidence bearing on every aspect of health and health care — and consulted widely with experts and citizens from coast to coast to coast. From his focus on the values that Canadians hold near and dear, Romanow concluded that the model of publicly funded health insurance can and must be preserved, and, furthermore, that it should be extended to encompass a wider range of "medically necessary" services. He proposed immediate coverage for those facing high ("catastrophic") drug costs and those in need of home care because they are mentally ill, because they have just been discharged from hospital or because they require palliative care. Romanow also identified the need for greater accountability for the vast sums of money spent on health care. He recommended the drafting of a "covenant" with Canadians and the establishment of an arm's-length health council responsible for safeguarding the terms of the covenant and for reporting to the public on health outcomes achieved throughout the country. He pointed out the absolute necessity of developing vastly improved systems of health information management and of developing clear and far-sighted policies on the education and deployment of health human resources, access to care (particularly for Aboriginal populations and in remote, rural and small-town Canada) and safeguarding the quality of care. It was Romanow's conclusion as well that the adoption of multidisciplinary practices offering a range of primary-care services "24/7" is central to the transformation and sustainability of the system, as is integration of its many discrete elements/service providers.

The sixth and final volume of the report of the Senate committee's two-year study of the state of health care in Canada appeared a month before the Romanow report. Sweeping and thorough in scope, the report by Senators Kirby and LeBreton and their colleagues added to the consensus that emerged from the four provincial bodies. The Senate committee did differ in some respects from Romanow, notably with regard to the need for additional sources of financing, the role of competition among public- and private-sector providers in achieving increased productivity, the particular needs and roles of hospitals, the wisdom of reopening the *Canada Health Act* and the workability of what it called a "Care Guarantee" to deal with dangerously long waits for service. On the whole, however, there was agreement on the majority of key policy issues — the need for stronger leadership/governance; better health information management; more accountability; greater integration of the system's players; a longer-term, more policy-driven approach to the education and training of health professionals; interdisciplinary teamwork and changes in the rules to permit every profession and discipline to provide the full scope of services warranted by the education, training and experience of its members; extended coverage of publicly funded health care, which would include, at least partially, the costs of prescription drugs and home care; and the central requirement of a dramatic change in the provision of primary care, creating a service available locally at all hours, day and night, from teams of providers offering the range of services needed to maintain good health and restore good health to those affected by commonplace illnesses and non-life-threatening injuries.

Six and eight years later, the problems and challenges addressed by the Senate committee and the Royal Commission were the same as those that faced Ontario's Health Services Restructuring Commission in 1996. If anything, most were made more intractable by the passage of time and deeper entrenchment of the resistance to change. Similarly, the reception of policy recommendations for fundamental change and the strategies to implement them — by governments and by organizations with a vested interest in the health care system — has remained cool, whether in Ontario, Quebec, Saskatchewan, Alberta or Canada as a whole. Daunting as the policy environment seemed to the Ontario commissioners when they set out, the fact is that the trail they broke touched nearly all the bases later covered by the other provincial pioneers and by Senator Kirby et al. and Commissioner Romanow. The way is blazed to a much brighter future for health care than will be reached by merely adding more and more money in a doomed attempt to maintain the status quo. It remains, however, for governments, the funders of health care, the care providers in all their diversity and the concerned people of Canada to summon up the courage to change the policy framework around health care and take that trail.

NOTES

1. Conference Board of Canada, as quoted in Standing Senate Committee (2002a).
2. Published in 1974, the Lalonde report, *A New Perspective on the Health of Canadians*, was the first major government report to suggest that health services are not the chief determinant of health. (Marc Lalonde was federal minister of health and welfare.)
3. Dr. Michael Gordon, National Advisory Council on Aging, as quoted in Standing Senate Committee (2002a, 5).
4. Described in Standing Senate Committee (2002a, 7).
5. Standing Senate Committee (2002a, 9).
6. Computed tomography and magnetic resonance imaging.
7. The other "winds" are new ideas and ways of doing things, chip-driven technology and financial pressures.
8. Bill C-6, *Personal Information Protection and Electronic Documents Act*, passed on April 13, 2000.
9. In 1996, the average age of Canada's Aboriginal population was 25.5 years, 10 years younger than the general population.
10. McEwan and Goldner (2000), cited in Standing Senate Committee (2002a).
11. The Heseltine report, *Towards a Blueprint for Change: A Mental Health Policy and Program Perspective* (1983); the Graham report, *Building Community Support for People: A Plan for Mental Health in Ontario* (1988); *Putting People First: The Reform of Mental Health Services in Ontario* (1993); and *Implementation Planning Guidelines for Mental Health Reform* (1994). All of these strongly endorsed the principle of moving mental health care from psychiatric hospitals into the community, where people with mental illness could receive the services they needed when required.
12. Mazankowski (2001). The Clair Commission sat from June to December 2000, the Fyke Commission from June 2000 to April 2001, and the Mazankowski Council from August 2000 to January 2002.

CHAPTER 3

VOLUNTARY GOVERNANCE

Ontario's public hospitals, like most in Canada, have a long history of dependence on the voluntary governance of private citizens drawn from the communities they serve.

Notwithstanding the term *public*, few public hospitals in Ontario are owned and governed by government, whether municipal, provincial or federal. Until it was recommended by the HSRC that they be divested, Provincial Psychiatric Hospitals were the only hospitals actually owned, governed and operated by the Government of Ontario. The owners of most hospitals are independent, private organizations, generally not-for-profit corporations registered provincially or federally. Their members are usually volunteers from the community served by the hospital who have responded to a public notice with an application for membership and have paid a small annual fee. A large number of hospitals that offer both acute and continuing care are "faith-based" — that is, owned by religious organizations, the majority by orders of Roman Catholic sisters or the church's successor organization, the Catholic Health Corporation of Ontario. A few hospitals are owned by municipal governments. A very small number, all small and highly specialized, are privately owned for-profit hospitals that qualify as "public" because their services are offered to the public and they are funded out of the public purse on the same terms as not-for-profit hospitals.

Leadership or governance of Ontario's public hospitals is usually provided by a board of directors (or governors or trustees) elected or appointed annually by the organization's owners at their annual general meeting. These boards, like the hospital corporations themselves, are usually made up of volunteers drawn from and representative of the community, district or region served by the hospital. The hospital's president, executive director or chief executive officer (the manager in charge, employed by the board) is also a board member. Other board members include representatives of physicians with what are called "privileges"[1] in the hospital and representatives of its employees. The board's membership and modus operandi are set out in the bylaws of each public hospital corporation and are subject to the general requirements of Ontario's *Public Hospitals Act*.

The work of the HSRC was of great interest and, more often than not, concern to the board of every public hospital and its senior management. Not only are hospitals integral to the health care system, they are also important contributors to the local economy. Any questioning of their future is perceived by most people not only as a threat to their preferred means of accessing health care but as a threat to the community itself. Consequently, during the unsettling times when the HSRC was restructuring hospitals, the public's anxiety and demand for timely information was reflected by hospital board members in their capacity as both members of the board and concerned members of the community. This anxiety was also given expression in the concerns of municipal governments and other organizations representative of the affected population.

Although nominally and legally in charge in every respect, hospital boards in Ontario have, over the years, become accustomed to more and more second-guessing if not direction by bureaucrats in the Ministry of Health. The propensity of bureaucrats to intrude on hospital governance and management has developed over many years in response to government concern at the rate of growth of hospitals' publicly funded budgets. The leash was also shortened as successive governments took more and more heat, especially in the media, for increasingly long waiting lists and other problems with what came to be referred to as a provincial "hospital system." Another factor was that government funding became the predominant component of hospital financing, displacing such sources of revenue as private fundraising or fee for services (private accommodation, for example) not covered by public health insurance. Consequently, dealing with government through the Ministry of Health has become a process both familiar and stressful to hospital boards and especially their senior managers.

The HSRC burst on the scene as a new player possessed of enormous power over the present and future — and even the very existence — of institutions cherished in their communities and ferociously defended by their boards, managers, physicians and employees. Nothing like the commission had ever been seen before. A good deal of the concern of each board and its chief executive officer arose from having to figure out whether this new player presented a threat or an opportunity and, whatever the case, how to deal with it. For many boards, establishment of the HSRC forced them to confront, often for the first time, just what their responsibilities were as governors. Their institutions, in addition to having become almost totally dependent on the province for funding, were being transformed from their traditional and legal "stand alone" status by the expectation that they join a nascent but growing "hospital system." Once independent, they were expected to be increasingly interdependent. This concept of governance could be rather frightening, even overwhelming, especially to the boards of smaller hospitals.

Governance is synonymous with leadership and is coupled with accountability both for its effectiveness and for the performance of the organization. Governance has to do primarily with the vitally important process of creating the vision and mission of the enterprise — what it will be and what it will do — as well as defining the goals and objectives it must meet in order to achieve the vision and mission. Governance includes articulating the values of the organization and its owners and the policies that derive from these values — policies on the choices that its members must make in order to achieve the desired outcomes. It also entails putting in place the management necessary to achieve those outcomes and evaluating the performance of managers and the organization. Among the tools of governance are influence, direction, planning, funding, incentives, penalties and rules. It is with governors that "the buck stops." Governors are accountable to the owners of the enterprise and those who benefit from it. They are not and should not try to be managers.

Management, or administration, is different from governance. Whereas governance has to do with *what* is to be done in accordance with definite *values*, management has to do with *how* policies are implemented and how things are done by and within the organization. Management is an executive function with authority for the operational control and direction of activities. It requires and employs a wide range of both general and specialized skills and the expertise and experience necessary to design and direct the organizational structure, budgeting and operational planning, finances, human and physical resources, internal and external communication, record keeping, evaluation of progress — the full range of activities in which an organization engages to achieve its desired outcomes. Managers are accountable to governors.

Accountability, on the part of both governors and managers, is the process of being held responsible. It includes evaluating how well the organization's actions serve to achieve the desired and measured outcomes, in both the short and the long term. Governors' ultimate accountability to the organization's owners and those it serves is for the effectiveness of their leadership, primarily for progress over the intermediate and long term toward realization of the organization's vision, adherence to its values and achievement of its mission; it includes holding its managers accountable for their performance. The accountability of managers relates to the effectiveness with which they direct the organization toward its desired outcomes, ensure that its members adhere to and exemplify its values, and see that its activities contribute effectively and efficiently to implementation of its operating plan and achievement of its goals and objectives.

It is fair to say that the vast majority of the governors of Ontario's 225 public hospitals had only a vague appreciation of these concepts when the HSRC began its work in 1996. The situation is likely not much different today except for the higher proportion of large, consolidated urban hospitals created by the commission. Generally speaking, the larger the hospital the greater the effort made to educate its board about the concepts of governance, management and accountability and to evaluate each member's performance and contribution to the board and institution. Characteristically, the boards of large hospitals have higher expectations of their members; most distinguish clearly between governance and management processes and evaluate the effectiveness of both. But do the boards of large hospitals generally provide more effective governance than those of small ones? Are they more accountable? It is hard to tell when hospital decision-making is so heavily influenced by the Ministry of Health.

The tradition of voluntary governance began in the days when hospitals were entirely local, providing care only to people living in the community in which the hospital was located and the immediate area. The boards of such hospitals served two functions: to ensure that the hospital was aware of and met, as far as possible, the needs of the people it served; and to represent the hospital in the community and strengthen the idea of its belonging to that community, regardless of who actually owned it. Although diminished today by virtue of referrals to specialists elsewhere and the easy transport of patients to hospitals far and wide, these two functions continue to dominate the work of hospital boards, especially in small and mid-sized rural and remote communities. In fact the HSRC found that these "local" functions applied to most urban hospitals as well, even some very large ones offering sophisticated services to a population drawn from the whole province and beyond.

The great strength of voluntary governance is that it is based on the selfless commitment of people who care enough about the hospital that serves their community, district or region to volunteer their time and energy, together with their expertise, experience and reputation, to participate in its operation. Such people will also know a good deal about their communities and the needs of its members for hospital services, an invaluable resource when matching resource allocation with community needs. Service on a hospital board is also a good training ground, albeit sometimes abused, for those interested in elected office and other kinds of community service.

The downside is the propensity of local boards to be parochial, focused on the affairs and welfare of their own hospital and community to the exclusion of all else. The idea of working with other hospitals is a tough sell to the members of such hospital boards (and their managers) — those who genuinely believe that anything that compromises the autonomy of their institution or community poses a threat. They feel greatly threatened by the concept of their hospital being interdependent, even when such interdependence — for laundry, food, financial, purchasing or managerial services, for example — could save money for reallocation to clinical programs.

The survival instincts of organizations are as strong as those of individuals. They come quickly to the fore in the face of threats, real or imagined, and once aroused are not easily overcome by a hospital board or, especially, an "outside" change agent like the HSRC. The HSRC knew from the outset that this would be one of its greatest challenges; there was never any doubt that the end result of hospital restructuring would be more interdependence among hospitals, even consolidation of hospitals into larger, integrated units.

To be fair, not all hospital boards were opposed to this concept; a few had moved in advance of the commission's establishment to implement it. The Toronto General and the Toronto Western had merged in the mid-1980s to form the Toronto Hospital (along with Princess Margaret Hospital, they now form the University Health Network). In London, Victoria and University Hospitals had merged. In Windsor, the Metropolitan General and Windsor Western had merged to form the Windsor Regional Hospital, and the Salvation Army Grace and the Hôtel Dieu had combined forces in an alliance that, for most purposes, made the two hospitals function as one. But these were exceptions. The rule was to protect autonomy at all costs. The common strategy was to do as little as possible as slowly as possible to accommodate what most boards saw as unreasonable attacks on the independence of their institutions, attacks they considered to be darkly cloaked in politically correct rhetoric about the need to build "networks" and "integrated systems." Many hospital boards perceived the networks and systems being discussed as nothing more than cunningly camouflaged threats even to the continued existence of their hospitals. Naturally, the survival instinct became a powerful underlying factor in every discussion.

FAITH-BASED HOSPITALS

Nowhere was that instinct more highly developed than among the owners and governors of Ontario's faith-based hospitals — Catholic, Jewish, Salvation Army and Seventh-Day Adventist. Of these, the largest number by far were Catholic hospitals, many located in mid-sized communities that were also home to a somewhat larger secular hospital. In two-hospital towns, the history of the relationship between the two institutions was frequently one of uneasy mutual tolerance that, at best, extended to watchful collaboration in a few selected programs. In a few cases, however — in the absence of planning or other leadership, and in the face of continued financial constraints — hospitals had risen to the challenge and found ingenious ways to "do more with less" in collaboration with a neighbouring secular or faith-based hospital. At worst, though, the history was one of open competition for staff (especially specialist physicians and surgeons), equipment, charitable giving in the community, clinical programs and, above all, public recognition, approbation and loyalty. Creation of the HSRC was a clear signal that in most if not all such communities the long-standing status quo would soon come to an end; only one hospital would remain. Catholic hospitals in particular perceived the commission as a threat to their very survival.

Notwithstanding all other considerations, two issues quickly became central — providing governance to hospitals in pursuit of their Catholic mission, and providing the community with reproductive services, specifically abortions and related services that ran counter to the fundamental values and teaching of the Roman Catholic Church. Other important matters proved amenable to ingenuity and compromise, matters such as developing ways to ensure genuine representation of the community on boards of directors that, in the end, were appointed by the religious orders, who still owned most Catholic hospitals. But it was clear from the outset to the commission, to the owners and governors of all Catholic hospitals and to members of the communities potentially affected that it was going to be difficult if not impossible to get around the fact that these faith-based hospitals could countenance neither mergers with secular institutions nor the provision, in their institutions, of completely legal abortions and related services that were demanded by and needed in the communities concerned.

From day one, therefore, the Catholic Health Association of Ontario (CHAO) and its membership had a number of reasons to fear the commission. Three of these reasons were central. The HSRC was apparently resolved and empowered to make a choice between hospitals in two-hospital towns and cities, putting an end to both competition and long-standing, carefully worked out rapprochements that had preserved a respected role for each. If the commission's stark choice was the Catholic hospital, that institution would be forced to confront the most unwelcome question of how to meet the community's need for abortion and related services. Finally, control over who sat on the hospital's board could no longer rest exclusively with the institution's owners; it would have to be shared with the community at large.

From the outset of the HSRC's mandate, the CHAO expressed a number of concerns about the *Savings and Restructuring Act* and the role of the commission — namely, that:

> the unrestricted powers conferred on the minister by the Act were much too broad
> delegation to the HSRC of the power to close and amalgamate hospitals removed accountability for the consequences of such decisions from elected officials
> the possibility of amalgamation or merger with nondenominational hospitals constituted a threat to the mission of Catholic hospitals
> the possibility of the HSRC's ordering Catholic hospitals to provide abortion and related services or to cease providing other services also constituted a threat to their mission
> if Catholic hospitals amalgamated or merged with nondenominational hospitals, a loss of assets was possible
> adequate representation on the governing body of amalgamated or merged hospitals could not be assured

The commission recognized and was sensitive to these concerns, especially those related to its ordering the amalgamation of Catholic and secular hospitals. Representatives of the CHAO were very clear in their advice that such mergers ran counter to canon law, the body of ecclesiastic decrees derived from papal and council pronouncements to which the Church and its adherents are bound. The same interpretation was provided by other authorities, both religious and secular, that the HSRC consulted in Canada and elsewhere. In other respects canon law was thought by most authorities to provide sufficient flexibility to permit consideration of a variety of alternatives to the status quo. On the question of amalgamation with a secular organization, however, it was narrowly and firmly cast. The commission therefore essentially took this option off the table as a means of continuing the proud tradition of separate secular and religious hospitals, a tradition that, in many communities, it would have preferred to preserve in one merged institution. Only two options remained:

> to have the hospitals concerned form a Joint Executive Committee (JEC), a body made up of representatives of the boards of two or more hospitals with the authority to make operational decisions to facilitate integration of their services and programs and their clinical, professional and administrative personnel
> to order one of the hospitals to cease operations and to close

This short list was further constrained by the CHAO's opposition to JECs, or at best its undisguised lack of enthusiasm for them. The CHAO's spokesmen believed the concept would also compromise the mission of Catholic hospitals, less so than forced mergers perhaps, but sufficiently to preclude its consideration. Had the commission ignored that opposition and ordered the formation of JECs between Catholic and secular hospitals in two-hospital communities, the hospitals concerned and the CHAO may well have acquiesced, in the end, and participated in their formation. But it was the HSRC's considered opinion that forced or even grudging collaboration would provide neither the hospital nor the community with the committed leadership needed to face the challenges ahead. So, apart from those few examples in which JECs or their equivalent between a Catholic and a secular hospital were proposed as part of local solutions,[2] canon law and the views of the CHAO left the commission with only one bleak option: to order one of the restructured institutions to close.

That is not to say that this situation prevailed only between faith-based and secular hospitals. In several communities the commission encountered boards that were, from the beginning, implacably opposed even to considering the formation of a JEC and, for that matter, any device to effect collaboration much less integration with another hospital. Here, too, recognizing the ineffectiveness of any forced partnership, the commission opted, in most cases, to close one hospital and transfer its assets to the one that it considered better equipped to meet the needs of the community.

GOVERNANCE MODELS

The HSRC realized early on that if there was a single key to success in hospital restructuring, it was governance. Indeed governance/leadership is the central element in successful change anywhere, certainly in every constituent provider of health services, be it hospitals, home care, mental health care or primary care. Without leadership by deeply committed people with their eyes firmly fixed on a shared vision, nothing of lasting benefit will result.

Appreciating the fact that governance could be either a force for or a barrier to change, the commission formulated a series of principles to guide its exploration and discussion of alternative approaches to and models of governance. Its goal was to ensure that the governance models adopted by the hospitals and communities it restructured, however different from one another they might prove to be, would all produce leadership that would be a reliable and resolute force for rather than a barrier to change. It was critical that the HSRC find approaches and structures appropriate for the institutions and communities concerned, establishing new leadership and making it quickly operational. The first, vital step for each newly created hospital corporation was to define its future, a key governance responsibility. The commission's guiding principles were:

> > The tradition of voluntary governance has served Ontario's hospitals and their communities well over the past many decades. Preferably this form of governance should be adhered to and enhanced in a restructured hospital sector and more broadly in a restructured health system.
> > Significant benefit has been and should continue to be derived from the diversity of traditions and cultures that exists within the hospital sector and throughout the many constituents of the health system in Ontario. One size does not and cannot fit all.
> > Important as that principle is, however, the maintenance of individual traditions and cultures must not stand in the way of progressively greater collaboration among hospitals and between them and other providers of health care services. Maintaining difference in tradition and

culture cannot trump the shift from autonomy to interdependence — that essential step toward the goal of providing high-quality patient care more efficiently effectively and with more seamless continuity.
> Given the fragmented nature of the so-called system, priority must be given to the creation of governance structures and functions that promote interdependencies among hospitals and between hospitals and other providers. It is only out of such interdependencies that a genuine health services *system* can be built and maintained.
> There is no one best model of governance or leadership that can be applied across the many and diverse communities of Ontario. In searching out different models to serve that diversity, the overarching criterion should be that each will promote increased integration of hospitals and of hospitals with other elements of the system and optimize efficiency and effectiveness throughout.
> New governance models should facilitate both greater integration of institutions and their activities *and* maintenance (or enhancement) of the distinctiveness of each individual participating institution and organization. In other words, it should permit hospitals (and others) to have the best of both worlds — to retain their identities and also be team players.
> The search for the best alternative governance structure to fit the circumstances of a given institution, organization, community, district or region is best conducted by those who will be most affected — people on the ground. Locally developed solutions are preferable to those imposed from the outside, whether by the commission or anybody else.

A draft and explanation of these principles was aired publicly for the first time in a speech given by the commission's chair to the annual meeting of the CHAO on September 26, 1996, six months after the HSRC had been formed. Sinclair concluded:

> Governance, as a structure, as a process, and as a symbol, is not a problem unless the imperatives of separate governance, the imperatives of so-called autonomy, stand in the way of system building and coming quickly to rational, amicable solutions to the puzzle of how best to organize the institutional and organizational resources of the elements of the so-called system into a real system. (Sinclair 1966)

During the weeks and months leading up to this meeting, the commission had pondered the many unknowns of governance — its concept, forms, approaches, structures and functions. The debate revolved around a series of questions:

> What are the best ways in which to approach the design of a system of governance in order to achieve the goals of a horizontally integrated hospital sector?

> Should the governance of hospitals be centralized (as in Alberta's Regional Health Authorities) or decentralized (distributed among individual hospitals, as in Ontario)? What are the theoretical and observed advantages and disadvantages of a single board for an entire hospital sector, region or province?

> Would stronger governance structures in hospitals enhance or inhibit the collective development of standards and practices, as in, for example, information management or human resources?

> Would these enhance or inhibit vertical integration with other forms of health care such as home care or long-term care?

> What actions, taken either locally or centrally (by the HSRC or the ministry), would help local governance to achieve greater integration among hospitals in its community, district or region, and to build stronger relationships with other providers of health services?

The commission's debate on these questions culminated in development of the principles, first described in the chair's speech to the CHAO, that guided the HSRC as it proceeded with hospital restructuring, community by community. From the outset the commission had no preconceived notions, much less the narrow prescription that some people later claimed it had, of the governance options it was prepared to accept. The HSRC was genuinely open to all manner of proposals from the communities concerned, provided they fit within the broad envelope of principles. Subsequent claims that the HSRC had developed, or had been given by the government, a small menu of acceptable governance options, from which it was not prepared to accept much if any deviation, were simply unfounded. It is true that when phase I was completed a relatively narrow range of options was selected among the many hospitals and communities affected by restructuring. But that narrow range was not preordained; the options evolved from the HSRC's own reviews and its response to solutions proposed locally to meet the needs and challenges that the commission and the hospital governors and managers encountered, community by community. They were the options the commission believed could provide restructured hospitals and their communities, districts and regions with the leadership required in today's world.

In the end, the governance options chosen by the commission came down to six:[3]

> full amalgamation or merger of two or more hospitals into a new corporate entity separate from the entities of its founding members
> full amalgamation or merger of two or more hospitals with the requirement that the new governance continue to be advised on specific issues for a specified period by a subsidiary board or standing committee
> agreement on an alliance between the separate boards of two or more hospitals to combine a wide range of specified activities through consolidation of funding, administrative, clinical and/or support services without creating a new corporation
> formation of a JEC made up of representatives of the separate boards of two or more hospitals empowered to make decisions relating to integration of specified aspects of the administrative and clinical operations of the participating institutions
> a series of specific contracts between the separate boards of two or more hospitals specifying in detail their agreement to collaborate in specified activities, the rights and duties of each party, and remedies and penalties associated with any breach of the contract
> closure of a hospital with relinquishment of its governance (and possibly ownership), management and operations to another hospital corporation

Only two options applied to the commission's recommendations to the minister on the formation of networks of rural and northern hospitals:

> "cluster" boards to facilitate the collaboration of several separate boards, together with JECs and other joint structures (including shared management)
> contractual agreements (comparable to the fifth multiple-contract option described above) setting out how the networked hospitals would work together with respect to clinical services, support services, and management and administration

Looking back on the results in aggregate, the commission ordered the application of various approaches to hospital governance, utilizing all the options variably, depending on its assessments of local circumstances and taking into account solutions developed locally. There were only three rules. The first was that every solution to provide a restructured hospital or group of hospitals with governance adhere to the commission's established (and advertised) principles. The second was, in effect, an additional principle taken from the report of the task force on the *Public Hospitals Act* on which both Mark Rochon and Duncan Sinclair had served in the early 1990s. It was that hospital boards not be "captured" by any constituency but be genuinely and generously representative of the population of the community, district or region served. Accordingly, all *Notices* and *Directions* issued by the HSRC to hospitals included the following statement: "The governance structure (of the board) must be representative of the communities served and have regard to the demographic, linguistic, cultural, economic, geographic, ethnic, religious, and social characteristics of the (community) region." The third rule had to do with the commission's concern that hospital boards not be naive with respect to the realities and complexities facing contemporary institutions. In all cases where new boards were being created (i.e., through amalgamation of previously separate organizations), the commission issued an additional directive: "That governance plans ensure that members of the new Board have relevant experience and expertise."

It was of great concern to the commission that patients and populations dependent on clinical programs being transferred from one hospital to another not fall through the cracks or find those programs demoted to low priority by the recipient hospital. In cases where it saw the possibility of that happening, the HSRC issued specific *Directions* that the hospital's governance be amended to provide the necessary protection. In a few cases, very specific *Directions* were issued to ensure that the boards of long-established hospitals were enlarged to reflect their responsibility for particular programs transferred from other hospitals. For example, with respect to the transfer of HIV-AIDS and other programs from Wellesley-Central Hospital, the board of St. Michael's Hospital was ordered to appoint, for a period of three years, one-third of its members from a list of candidates provided by Wellesley-Central's board. And Doctors Hospital, which was ordered to transfer its community-oriented and other programs to what was then the Toronto Hospital,[+] had to appoint three members of its board to the board of the Toronto Hospital and to constitute itself as an advisory committee to that hospital for a period of up to two years.

COMMUNITY PROCESS

Consolidation of hospital governance was the most immediate outcome of the HSRC's hospital restructuring work in most of Ontario's urban centres. This first step in unified governance or leadership was key to what followed, bringing together the hospitals' senior administration, other administrative and support services and, finally, clinical programs.

This was easier said than done. Consolidating often fiercely separate governing boards made for a difficult, unnatural and extremely "bumpy" transition for communities and their hospitals. If it occurred at all, it was a transition that would have been interminable without the intervention of experienced facilitators to lay the ground, drive the process of negotiation, mediate disputes when necessary and do everything else needed to help the parties, as the saying goes, "get to yes."

Whenever possible, acting on the principle that locally derived solutions are preferable to all others, the commission focused its *Directions* on *what* was to be done — the goals and objectives to be achieved. It preferred to leave the method of achieving them to the people concerned, those on the ground. To facilitate the negotiation of *how* things would be done, the HSRC appointed facilitators experienced in such matters to help the people develop approaches and solutions appropriate for their particular circumstances. Although the process was in many cases long, tedious and difficult, in most communities it did produce local solutions that represented hard-won but genuine consensus among the players and that required, in the end, only the commission's endorsement. There were a few failures, of course, but even in the absence of consensus the local negotiations usually produced strong majority positions that carried local "buy in" sufficiently for the HSRC to feel justified in imposing them on the community.

The people acting in the role of facilitator were selected and appointed by the HSRC after it had asked the hospitals concerned for nominees and had secured agreement from each as to the acceptability of the appointee. In those communities where the relationship among the hospitals concerned was characterized by rivalry compounded by distrust, facilitation began with groundwork as basic as developing and getting agreement on a process to identify and reduce the barriers to a better relationship.

Often, history was the major roadblock, reinforced by inaccurate recollection of events long past and the attribution of the motives behind them, which were made malevolent by time. In a few cases, simple civic rivalry between adjacent towns was enough to jeopardize restructuring options that everybody agreed were needed desperately in the district — "but located there, not here!" One unhappy intervener told the commission that he would never travel on a particular Air Canada flight because that was the one the minister of municipal affairs had taken many years before to announce the amalgamation of Port Arthur and Fort William into the new community of Thunder Bay.

Another common problem in amalgamations between small and large hospitals was that the smaller partner perceived a takeover while the larger one perceived loss of control over the greater asset base it brought to the union. In the communities where they were appointed, the facilitators were indispensable to the establishment of trust among the players. Without their expertise, experience and reputation for even-handedness, hospital restructuring would have been delayed even longer in many communities.

One of the immediate outcomes of restructuring in most urban centres was the consolidation of hospitals, initially their governance and subsequently their senior administration. The first step in achieving restructured governance was to explore opportunities for consolidating administrative and support services and clinical programs. In many communities the consolidation of governance would not have been possible without the appointment of facilitators to lay the groundwork and assist the parties in implementing the HSRC's *Directions*.

Toward the end of its mandate the commission convened a meeting of all facilitators[5] to discuss their experiences and to draw out the lessons they had learned, community by community. There was broad agreement on a number of conditions that were either prerequisites to or enablers of a process leading to effective leadership. The first condition was the HSRC's legal authority to impose its will, if necessary. It permitted the facilitators to pose what proved in every case to be a rhetorical question: "Would you rather do this yourself (develop for your hospital an effective governance that reflects your understanding of what will work in your community) or have the commission do it for you?" In other words, "If you don't do it, the HSRC will!" Related to that was the understanding that what was being negotiated in each community was *how* the commission's *Directions* were to be implemented. The *Directions* themselves were not negotiable. On that the HSRC had declared itself to be intransigent. In addition, the government had made it clear that it would not interfere with any of the commission's decisions. There was no way to get around the commission except in the courts, and then only on the grounds of faulty process. The facilitators were able to set a ground rule from the outset: "We are here not to talk about *what* to do, only to talk about how to get it done."

Another condition was that the facilitators be entirely neutral throughout and that this be clear to all parties; their sole responsibility was to facilitate a mutually satisfactory agreement as quickly as possible. It was also seen as important that the commission remain detached from the delicate processes established to negotiate the terms of reference for the discussions. These included the parties' expectations regarding the communication of the various positions being considered, how issues were being resolved and what the next steps would be. Although removed from the process of negotiation itself, the facilitators agreed that it was critical they retain the right and responsibility to make their own recommendations to the HSRC (and that the HSRC take these seriously) if the parties could not agree or if the discussions were proceeding too slowly. In effect this condition meant that in extremis the facilitator could act as an arbitrator whose decisions would be taken by the HSRC as binding. Finally, it was viewed as crucial that the HSRC be prepared to provide facilitators with support when needed — for example, by attending a meeting in the community to discuss a particular direction or to stress the importance of meeting deadlines for agreement on matters under negotiation.

LESSONS LEARNED

The commission learned a number of important lessons from the amalgamations or mergers of hospitals that it ordered throughout Ontario.

One such lesson was that a firm foundation had to be laid for the new board to take over responsibility from the boards of the pre-existing hospitals. It had to be made clear that the new organization had exclusive authority and that the contributions of the hospitals' founders, though remembered, valued, respected and honoured, were in the past. It was essential that the methods used to nominate, select and appoint the new board members ensure their full commitment to the new hospital (and the perception of such). Although nominated from different constituencies identified as having distinct and often different interests in the new hospital, board members could certainly reflect those interests but could not be bound to represent them; once appointed to the board, their sole constituency was the hospital and the whole community it served.

Another lesson learned was the importance of developing, through the facilitation process, protocols and processes to ensure a smooth transition of governance from the pre-amalgamation boards to the new board. In addition to the legal steps necessary to transfer power, there were such matters as communicating to staff members, physicians, patients and the general public who was in charge and when they would be taking over. To avoid abrupt loss of valuable experience, in a number of communities members of the pre-amalgamation boards were invited to serve on committees or work on special projects set up by the new board to address matters related to the amalgamation or other issues of vital concern to the new hospital.

Although it proved critical for the new board to streamline the processes leading to the recruitment and appointment of its chief executive officer, it was apparent to the commission that the transition to a new set of internal processes and the development of a new board culture could not be rushed. A transition phase of two to three years is needed to develop and implement proactive strategies to build the new team as well as the confidence and competence necessary to provide effective governance. Mentoring within the new board can contribute to the implementation of those processes. So too can the development of open communication between the board and the new management team.

Among high-priority tasks are community liaison and the establishment of a foundation to raise funds, perhaps even a capital campaign to support new construction. There are many such tasks to engage profitably a new hospital's owners, governors, managers and staff, all on behalf of the community served.

The establishment of JECs has worked well in areas where organizations had been jointly involved previously and where the different roles and responsibilities of each organization were clear. Issues that arose with respect to the roles of JECs had to do with uncertainty about whether these governance entities were permanent or temporary; uncertainty about whether their responsibilities related strictly to planning or included decision-making; difficulties in agreeing on appropriate membership and composition; the need for clarification concerning relationship and accountability to parent boards; and the barriers presented by the time, process and resources required to put into operation and legitimize the work of the JEC.

The fact remains that governance is central to successful change. If the leadership is right, all else will follow. If it is not, and if consensus among those who are supposed to lead is elusive or grudging, progress toward restructuring hospitals (or anything else) will be painfully slow.

Appendix 2
DEFINITIONS OF GOVERNANCE STRUCTURES

Term/definition	Essential elements
Amalgamation Two or more separate hospital corporations joining together and continuing as one corporation in accordance with the provisions of the *Corporations Act* and the *Public Hospitals Act*	• Results in a new corporate entity (i.e., a permanent structure with legal existence separate from that of its founders) • Must be in full compliance with provisions of the *Corporations Act* • Must receive approval of the minister of health, public guardian and trustee and Ministry of Consumer and Commercial Relations • Can result in one corporation absorbing the other or in the emergence of a merged corporation with new objects, arising out of the amalgamating corporation
Alliance agreement Two or more hospitals agree by contract to combine funding and management, clinical and/or support services to enhance quality and improve the delivery of hospital services through consolidation, *without creating a corporation*	• Created by way of a contract that might include the following: purpose and scope of the alliance; location of principal office; terms of the agreement; amount of capital contributions by each; accounting procedures and financial and other records; dissolution and liquidation; dispute-resolution mechanisms; management of the alliance, including the delegating of authority and responsibility for each participant
Joint Executive Committee (JEC) A body, comprising representatives of the governing boards of two or more participating hospitals, that has *authority to make decisions* on the operations of the participating hospitals in order to facilitate integration and linkages among hospitals, their services and programs and their clinical, professional and administrative personnel	• Participating hospitals continue to exist as separate entities, subject to *delegation* of certain authority to the JEC • Decision-making authority related to *specific issues* is explicitly delegated by the governing boards to the JEC • The relationship is created by way of a written agreement/contract that ideally sets out bylaws or protocols on the conduct of affairs and operations of the JEC, including accountability and reporting requirements with respect to governing boards • Requires the agreement of the majority of directors of each organization
Contract/agreement A written, legally enforceable document setting out the nature of the (integrated) relationship between two or more hospitals, including the contractual rights and duties of each party and any remedies and penalties for breach of such duties	• Meets the legal test for valid contract (e.g., offer, acceptance, consideration, consensus) • Sets out the exact contractual rights and duties of each party as well as remedies and penalties for breach thereof

Appendix 2
DEFINITIONS OF GOVERNANCE STRUCTURES (continued)

Term/definition	Essential elements
Relinquishment of operation and management A direction that the board of a hospital corporation relinquish operation, management and control (and in some instances ownership) of the hospital to another hospital corporation such that it ceases to be involved in the running of the hospital. The board of the hospital corporation to which operation, management and control is transferred assumes (subject to any direction to the contrary) sole responsibility for providing the programs and services of the hospital that is "relinquished" and for managing its resources and assets	• A "relinquishing" hospital is one that must give up the operation, management and control of some or all of its programs or services (and in some instances ownership) to another hospital • A "receiving" hospital is one to which the operation, management and control of programs or services (and in some instances ownership) are to be transferred from a relinquishing hospital

Appendix 3
HSRC-APPOINTED GOVERNANCE FACILITATORS

Facilitator	Assignment/communities
Tim Armstrong	**Haliburton, Kawartha and Pine Ridge** Assist with board structure changes for the Northumberland Health Care Corporation
Paul Cramer/Francine Pillemer	**Metro Toronto** Amalgamation of Orthopaedic and Arthritic Hospital, Sunnybrook Health Science Centre and Women's College Hospital
Michael Decter	**GTA/905** Amalgamation of Peel Memorial, Georgetown and District Memorial, and Etobicoke General **Kingston** Investigate potential of an interim agreement between Hotel Dieu, Kingston General Hospital and Providence Continuing Care Centre (working with Alan Hudson)
Michael Delaney	**Metro Toronto** Transfer of operation and management of programs and services of Doctors Hospital to the Toronto Hospital
Claude Halpin	**GTA/905** Amalgamation of Oakville Trafalgar Memorial and Milton General and District
Christine Hart	**Metro Toronto** Transfer of operation and management of Wellesley-Central to St. Michael's Hospital
Tom Heintzman	**Metro Toronto** Address resolution of outstanding issues regarding amalgamation of Orthopaedic and Arthritic Hospital, Sunnybrook Health Science Centre and Women's College Hospital
Alan Hudson	**Kingston** Investigate potential of an interim agreement between Hotel Dieu, Kingston General Hospital and Providence Continuing Care Centre (working with Michael Decter)

Appendix 3
HSRC-APPOINTED GOVERNANCE FACILITATORS (continued)

Facilitator	Assignment/communities
Hugh Kelly	**Metro Toronto** Develop a plan to transfer responsibility for the operation and management of programs and services at North York Branson to North York General **Pembroke** Develop a governance plan for Pembroke General
Graham Scott/Maureen Quigley	**GTA/905** Amalgamation of Whitby General Hospital, Oshawa General Hospital, North Durham Health Services and Memorial Hospital (Bowmanville) **Niagara** Amalgamation of St. Catharines General, Greater Niagara General, Welland County General, Shaver, Douglas Memorial, Niagara on the Lake, Niagara Rehabilitation Centre and Port Colborne General **Metro Toronto** Amalgamation of Addiction Research Foundation, Clarke Institute of Psychiatry, Donwood Institute and Queen Street Mental Health Centre Amalgamation of Toronto Rehabilitation Centre, Rehabilitation Institute of Toronto and Lyndhurst Hospital **Ottawa-Carleton** Amalgamation of Ottawa Civic, Ottawa General, Riverside and Salvation Army Grace **Sudbury** Amalgamation of Laurentian Hospital, Sudbury General and Memorial Hospital
Carolyn Sherk/Louise Leonard	**Metro Toronto** Transfer of operation and management of St. Bernard's Hospital to St. John's Rehabilitation Centre
Andrew Szende	**Metro Toronto** Amalgamation of Centenary Health Centre and Ajax Pickering General
Michael Watts	**Northeastern Ontario** Creation of a governance structure for the new Northeast Mental Health Centre

NOTES

1. The right to admit and treat patients.
2. In Lambton a Joint Operations and Planning Committee, single chief executive officer, management structure and medical advisory committee were proposed jointly by the Sarnia General Hospital, St. Joseph's Health Centre and Charlotte Eleanor Englehart Hospital.
3. See appendices 2 and 3 for details.
4. Now the University Health Network.
5. See appendix 4 for a list of HSRC-appointed facilitators.

CHAPTER 4

HOSPITAL RESTRUCTURING: THE COMMISSION'S POWER

It is only in recent times, at least in developed countries like Canada, that hospitals have become icons of health care. Until the advent of academic or science-based medicine, marked in North America by the Flexner report (Flexner 1910), hospitals were little more than sophisticated hostels, made so by their intensive staffing by nurses, doctors and others experienced in caring for the sick. People too sick or too badly injured to be looked after at home by family members and community physicians were put there, the majority of them to die in the compassionate care of the hospital's sponsors and staff members, many of them in religious orders.[1]

In some ways, hospitals are unchanged. They remain institutions of last resort, particularly large tertiary-care hospitals that provide a wide range of sophisticated services. They are expected to admit and provide care for patients whose illnesses cannot be diagnosed or treated confidently elsewhere or whose effective care requires specialized facilities and personnel available nowhere else. The hotel function that defined their early predecessors — in-patient care — still defines the hospital. A hospital's relative standing both among its peers and with the public remains largely determined by the number of beds it has — the more beds, the higher the status; although in recent years ambulatory services have been gradually earning hospitals recognition and respect as well.

Where today's hospitals differ most from those of the old days is that they are expected to rescue the great majority of their patients from life-threatening diseases and conditions. If admitted as in-patients, most patients (and their families) expect to leave the hospital alive and improved, if not well. Many more people than are admitted receive services in emergency rooms and outpatient clinics. Some are still admitted to die, but most people look to hospitals as safeguards, promoters and restorers of health, if not guarantors of high-quality health care in the communities in which they live.

It is easy to understand why, when medicare was introduced, priority was given to eliminating the financial barrier between hospital care and those who needed it. Hospitals provide care to the most acutely and gravely ill. They also constitute the single most expensive provider of health care, one that, before universal, publicly financed health insurance, presented the greatest threat to the financial survival of families with a sick member requiring more care than could be provided at home by the family and local general practitioner. Community-based nurses were rare; apart from those working in public health, nurses were trained and worked in hospitals. Ever since, even after public health insurance was extended to cover doctors' services, hospitals have been central to health care in Canada. In recent years they have become symbols of the health of health care itself.

The Health Services Restructuring Commission had to confront this iconic status in the first, hospital-restructuring, phase of its work, which occupied most of its attention from the spring of 1996 until well into 1999. It was this particular status of hospitals, their high community profile and the politically laden symbolism of "health of health care" associated with them that deterred successive governments from picking up the challenge of hospital restructuring in the 1980s and early 1990s. It led to the formation of the commission.

Iconic status or no, events — particularly adverse financial events — did not stand still during the 1980s and 1990s. They affected all publicly funded institutions as governments struggled to control public expenditures in the face of inflationary and other cost increases that outstripped the rate of growth of tax revenues. It was obvious to informed observers that Canada's public hospitals contained far more beds than were needed by the population, at least for acute-care services. Consequently, restructuring of a sort proceeded in Ontario, but covertly, as several successive governments used the blunt instrument of financial allocation — the "power of the purse." Year by year, funding increases were restricted to less than the rate at which hospitals' costs were increasing, not only labour costs but also capital costs and the associated operational cost of new technology — including, ironically, the diagnostic and other equipment that was enabling the rapid shift from in-patient to outpatient care. As for labour costs, as usual, pay raises took precedence over the number of people employed; nurses and other staff were laid off and beds were closed.

The development and availability of new knowledge and technology — new drugs, "keyhole" surgery and so forth — made it possible for hospitals to provide an ever-increasing proportion of their services safely and less expensively to patients on an ambulatory basis and to keep in-patients for much shorter stays; their throughput increased dramatically. Correspondingly, as the overall proportion of government funding allocated to hospitals continued to fall, spending on prescription drugs increased year by year and now is second only to hospital funding as a proportion of total (public and private combined) health care expenditures. The proportion spent on home care also continues to increase.

When the commission was established in 1996, the media's repeated reporting of more than 9,000 empty beds in Ontario and not a single hospital closure resonated with the public. Taxpayers could easily conceptualize what it cost them to maintain the equivalent of 30 to 35 empty mid-sized hospitals. Many people remembered a popular British television series from the early 1980s, *Yes Minister* (and its successor, *Yes Prime Minister*). One particularly humorous episode, "The Compassionate Society," featured the minister's incredulous and sharply querulous visit to a new, fully staffed, award-winning hospital that had yet to admit a single patient. Keeping open 30 to 35 empty hospitals, icons or not, struck most Ontarians as not a particularly sensible thing to do. It constituted inefficient use of resources; better to spend money on a reasonable number of hospitals that are full than on a vast number that are not.

Unlike the hospital in *Yes Minister*, however, Ontario's empty hospitals were not real; they were *virtual* hospitals, equivalent to real ones only by the mathematical conversion of their collections of empty beds into theoretical units of 300, the size of an average hospital. The empty beds were actually distributed hither and yon throughout all of the province's approximately 225 public hospitals. They took the form of unstaffed rooms, wards and sometimes wings, all unoccupied and out of sight but none — in the eyes of the general public — obviously redundant. In fact, there continued to be waiting lists for admission and, throughout this period, repeated media reports of people "waiting for a bed" in emergency-room corridors — reports that led the public to conclude that Ontario's hospitals had too few rather than too many beds. Informed observers knew, however, that if hospitals have the money to pay nurses, aides, cleaners and other workers, their beds will always be filled, accommodating patients who could certainly benefit from care of some kind. In the industry it is widely recognized that there is no such thing as an empty bed — only a bed that the hospital cannot afford to staff or to let its admitting physicians fill.

From a societal perspective, the question comes down to a cost-benefit analysis. How much benefit is derived from the high cost of care in an acute-care hospital bed relative to alternatives such as outpatient care or care by a family physician, nurse practitioner, or occupational or physical therapist, with the patient remaining at home or in a retirement or long-term-care facility? Obviously the results of that analysis depend upon many variables, including the acuity and severity of the patient's condition. Those with acute and severe problems benefit greatly from the intense and sophisticated care that acute-care hospitals provide. But for others the costs appear profligate when measured against the benefits either to the individual patient or to society. Another factor not frequently considered is that "Hospitals are dangerous places, especially if you do not need to be there!" (Fisher 2003)

Two approaches are used to conduct that cost-benefit analysis, one clinical and the other administrative. The clinical approach leaves it to attending physicians to decide whether their patients need the services provided in an acute-care bed. Patients who are judged not to need acute care are categorized as requiring an alternative level of care (ALC); their needs could be met in some other setting, such as at home with home care or in a rehabilitation or long-term-care facility, but a place at this alternative level is not immediately available. Basically, ALC patients are those waiting in hospital to go somewhere else. The reporting of ALC cases is a clinical decision that is entered in the patient's chart by the responsible or attending physician. The administrative approach to cost-benefit analysis is a collective one, based on the same individual clinical judgment. One simply compares the proportion of ALC patients in a given hospital with those of comparable hospitals and then seeks to explain any deviations.

Despite the 9,000 to 11,000 empty beds forced by cumulative budgetary stringency in the 1980s and 1990s, in 1996 Ontario's public hospitals continued to accommodate a high proportion of ALC patients. This led to the conclusion by informed observers that, provided additional alternative-care placements were to be made available (principally in home care, long-term care, rehabilitation, supportive housing and community support for patients with mental health problems), Ontario's public hospitals were, in aggregate, larger than necessary to meet the need for hospital-based acute care. Certainly this had been the new government's conclusion in 1995, when it formulated and implemented the two financial policy planks referred to earlier:

> funding of the health budget will remain constant over the period 1996-99
> funding of hospitals will be cut by 18 percent over the same period at a rate of 5, 6 and 7 percent annually[2]

Clearly focused on the magnitude and pace of the impending decrease in the funding of hospitals, the HSRC decided, at its initial meeting, to devote the first phase of its work to hospital restructuring and to concentrate on hospitals in the major cities and their suburbs. Each city encompassed several acute-care hospitals with records of collaboration that ranged from reasonable accommodation to overt resistance. In some cities, mergers had already taken place (Windsor, London and Sarnia) or were in the works (Toronto), making them fertile ground for the commission's early work. Eight municipalities — Hamilton, Kingston, London, Ottawa, Sudbury, Thunder Bay, Toronto and Windsor — accounted for the majority (65 percent) of spending on Ontario's hospitals.

DISTRICT HEALTH COUNCIL REPORTS

In each of these communities the relevant District Health Council had been at work for some time.[3] The reports of most DHCs contained credible restructuring options, with their recommendations buttressed by roughly comparable data and other information from the community concerned. From the outset, the HSRC was very much influenced by the DHC reports. Not only did its mandate include the explicit instruction to "take into account" the work and recommendations of the DHCs, but it also made great sense to do so. There was clear profit in the careful analytical work done by planners with firsthand experience of their communities' institutions and other providers of health care and in the time and effort the DHCs had devoted to local consultations. In its own modus operandi the HSRC relied heavily on those consultations; it decided at the outset not to duplicate them when forming its own judgment of each community's needs and wants when developing options for hospital restructuring, community by community.

Of all those reviewed by the HSRC, three DHC reports on hospital restructuring were exemplary — those for Thunder Bay,[4] Essex County and Metropolitan Toronto. The analysis of options they contained was comprehensive and the recommendations for redesign of the local hospital sector well supported by evidence drawn from the community. In all three communities, work had already begun to follow through on the DHC's recommendations, providing momentum on which the HSRC could build.

Thunder Bay

The Thunder Bay DHC began its review of the community's hospital services in 1992-93. Setting the stage was the fact that the five hospitals in the city, like hospitals everywhere, had been forced by financial constraints to make critical decisions relating to their staffing levels and the range of services they could provide. While some economies had been achieved, their independent decisions had not necessarily been the best from a system perspective; a number of identified gaps in service continued to be ignored. This challenge was similar to challenges faced elsewhere in the province, but the hospital agenda in Thunder Bay had to accommodate other complexities related to the geography of the region, population density, a shortage of specialists, duplication of some services and gaps in others, difficulties with patient access to highly specialized care, north/south tensions and the referral responsibilities of the city's hospitals for the whole of northeastern Ontario (Thunder Bay District Health Council 1994).

In its final report the DHC presented the series of options it had considered both for program realignment among the hospitals and for their governance. For the long term, it recommended that one site be developed for acute care and a second (existing) site be used for rehabilitation. Short-term strategies were developed to provide governance in common by consolidating the existing hospital boards and reducing the use of high-cost acute-care beds while providing lower-cost institutional and community-based alternatives.

Essex County

The *Final Report of the Steering Committee on Health System Reconfiguration* was approved by the Essex County DHC and accepted by the minister of health in February 1994, a full two years before the HSRC appeared on the scene. The report recommended consolidating the four Windsor hospitals onto two acute-care sites, closing the Salvation Army Grace Hospital and converting the Windsor Western Hospital into a long-term-care facility, a centre of excellence to provide some other regional services as well. The Leamington District and Memorial Hospital, 50 kilometres east of Windsor, serving south

Essex, western portions of Kent County and Pelee Island, was to develop a stronger role in ambulatory care and establish closer links to the hospitals in Windsor for in-patient care.

Partnership between the Hôtel Dieu and the Salvation Army Grace hospitals was approved in May 1994, followed in December by the merger of the Windsor Western and the Metropolitan General. By March 1996 the minister of health had approved $73 million in capital funding for redevelopment of the two consolidated hospital sites. This sum was deemed totally inadequate by the community, but it did represent the ministry's commitment to support locally developed restructuring plans at a time when the province was particularly short of money. During the previous year (September 1995) the DHC and the Windsor-Essex Health Unit had jointly published a health-status report on Essex County to provide additional information for use in planning the restructuring of hospitals and other health services.

Metropolitan Toronto

After two years of intensive research and public consultations, in late September 1995 the Metropolitan Toronto District Health Council (MTDHC) received the final report of its Hospital Restructuring Committee (HRC), *Directions for Change: Toward a Coordinated Hospital System for Metro Toronto*.[5] The MTDHC's hospital restructuring project had had three distinct phases. The first was analysis of the current size and capacity of Metro's hospital services and those deemed necessary to meet future needs. The second focused on options for reconfiguring the city's hospitals and culminated in the HRC's final report to the council. The third was a consultation phase seeking public input on the recommended options; the results were incorporated in the recommendations made in the HRC's final report. The MTDHC based its final report to the government on the need for significant, carefully planned change to effect restructuring of the hospital services available in Metropolitan Toronto. It set out specific recommendations for restructuring of hospitals throughout Metro, which were supported, in large part, by the hospitals that would be affected. It emphasized the need for reinvestment in community services and pointed out that service gaps, above and beyond those necessary to facilitate hospital restructuring (mental health, primary care, health promotion, long-term care, etc.), had to be addressed. It recommended that all savings realized from hospital restructuring be reinvested elsewhere, principally to increase the capacity of community-based health-service providers.

HEALTH INFORMATION

Notwithstanding all the empty, unstaffed beds in Ontario, one of the central questions before the commission as it faced the challenge of hospital restructuring was how many beds, and how much emergency and clinic capacity, were really needed, community by community. To confound the question, hospital beds fall into distinct categories, as the commissioners well knew. In addition to the acute-care beds that constitute the great majority in public hospitals, there are beds to accommodate patients with mental disorders, patients who require rehabilitation and patients with chronic conditions requiring longer-term hospitalization; this latter category, previously referred to as "chronic care," was redefined by the commission as "complex continuing care."

Although clues were available from comparisons of Ontario with other jurisdictions in Canada and elsewhere, the HSRC was aware that many factors bear on the calculation of a bed-to-population statistic — for example, the age, gender, health status and other characteristics of the population; length of stay in hospital; and the availability of alternative-care capacity. It concluded that while interjurisdictional comparisons were useful, they were too subject to uncontrolled and unmeasured variability to form a platform sufficiently robust to answer the question of how many beds were really needed. In fact, the commission realized early on that no mere calculation could yield a confident answer. In the first place, accurate and timely measures of many of the variables were simply unavailable. Secondly, some measures — health status, for example — are too subtle and complex to be captured reliably and reduced to a credible number in a "population-needs equation" by any known dispassionately objective method.

One of the HSRC's first challenges, which it met promptly and with a good deal of effort, was to acquire or gain access to a number of databases on the health care system in Ontario and to create useful linkages among them. The commission developed the most comprehensive integrated health database then extant in Ontario and probably in Canada. Nevertheless it was painfully clear that the health data available were inadequate for effective planning or most other purposes, including that of discharging accountability for resources spent on health care. The deficiencies were many and very serious. As this became increasingly obvious to the HSRC, the chair said so repeatedly in speeches to widely diverse audiences around the province:

> Despite the fact that the commission has as good or better [a] "handle" on the available health data and information than

anybody, if you asked me the perfectly reasonable question, "are we getting our money's worth?" I would have to answer, "I haven't a clue!" For the billions of dollars we are spending annually on health and health care, publicly and out of our own pockets, I can't even tell you how many individual interactions there have been in any year between those using and those providing health services; I have only fragmentary information about who (what providers) were involved; I don't know why each of those interactions took place or what went on, much less answer the most important question of all, "what, if any, benefit was the result?" The simple, sad fact is that we are attempting to govern and manage a multi-billion- dollar business using an information system that the owner of an ordinary corner store would consider seriously deficient. If the ordinary taxpayer had any idea how parlous is the state of the information available on our single most expensive and most highly cherished social program, s/he would have a fit! (Sinclair 2005)

It was small comfort to know that the capacity for health information management is not much better anywhere else in Canada or internationally.

If there is a redeeming virtue in this sorry state of affairs, it is that hospital data, at least those primarily related to in-patients, are by far the best of the lot. The HSRC turned its efforts to getting access to those data and to linking them to other relevant databases (such as census data). It used this information to develop what it referred to as "planning guidelines" and "benchmarks" that could be applied to the hospitals it had the power to restructure.

RESTRUCTURING METHODOLOGY

Given that the commission found nothing available elsewhere to import, the decision was taken to develop a made-in-Ontario approach to hospital restructuring. This rested on provincial policy guidelines where they existed[6] and on the principle of observed best practice where they did not. Three methodologies[7] were developed:

> a methodology for sizing and configuring the services of individual hospitals in relation to the patient populations they were being restructured

to serve. This methodology included best-practice benchmarks that the commission established for like categories of patient cases (Case Mix Groups[8]), which allowed comparison of the performance of different hospitals doing the same kind of work — caring for patients hospitalized for the same clinical conditions. In some cases best practice was defined by the average performance of hospitals in Ontario while in others the performance of the top 25 percent was used — that is, the 75th percentile.

> a methodology for forecasting to 2003 the needs of the community served for a spectrum of hospital services based on population and demographic projections by Statistics Canada and used by the Ontario Ministry of Finance. Those projections were modified by applying an expected-stay index to the predicted referral population to adjust for the anticipated acuity and/or complexity of individual visits. These forecasts were predicated on the hospital's achieving the utilization improvements identified by the previously applied sizing and configuration methodology.

> a funding/costing methodology for estimating the costs and savings associated with different restructuring options, to enable the HSRC to test its cost-effectiveness criterion and advise the minister how much implementation of its directions and recommendations would cost. It was based on application of the two other methodologies to the principal cost centres of hospitals: in-patient services, including operating and recovery rooms; ambulatory care related to the in-patient stay; clinical laboratories; diagnostic imaging; pharmacy; clinical nutrition; physical, occupational and other therapies; and food services.

The most carefully scrutinized (by the affected hospitals) of these methodologies was the first. Although there were some complaints (and recognition by the commission of the need for monitoring and adjustment in light of particular local circumstances), most hospitals accepted the 75th percentile as a reasonable target for what the HSRC identified as the key variable, length of stay, or the length of time patients with particular diagnoses remained in a hospital bed. By definition, many hospitals in Ontario had already achieved (and in some cases surpassed) that benchmark. The evidence was clear, however, that hospitals in many other jurisdictions were already meeting much more ambitious targets without a deleterious effect on the health of their populations.

As pointed out previously, the question of how many beds are needed is a complex one. But two factors predominate: the number of people in a given population admitted to a hospital bed, and the length of time each stays there. It was the length-of-stay variable that the commission held to most firmly as the foundation of its hospital sizing decisions. When a strong case was made, it did develop approaches to increase hospital capacity in relation to particular community needs, such as for joint-replacement or cardiac surgery or cancer services. But these adjustments were applied after the capacity of the hospital concerned had been decided — after applying the 75th percentile for length of stay by Case Mix Group.

In arriving at its sizing decisions, the commission also used software developed and adopted by the Ministry of Health, the Planning Decision and Support Tool. This tool had been developed to facilitate local and provincial comparisons of clinical efficiency among hospitals and assessment of their current utilization patterns and trends. It contained data and statistics applicable to most health care institutions in Ontario. Using it, the commission created benchmarks for utilization improvements that removed from hospitals' bed capacity that number related to 100 percent of their ALC patients and 100 percent of patients categorized as "avoidable admissions."[9] Where appropriate, the methodology also converted in-patient to outpatient surgery, again using the 75th percentile benchmark. The average length of stay was also adjusted against the 75th percentile. Both benchmarks were, as described, derived from the observed performance by hospitals with patients drawn from their respective catchment areas diagnosed with comparable conditions in 1995-96, the latest year for which the ministry and the commission had reliable data. On the basis of the observed data and application of the growth methodology, software was developed to define the likely catchment areas that would be served by restructured hospitals.

The commission's estimates of future growth in the need for hospital services were based on a methodology developed in 1996 by Ontario's Joint Policy and Planning Committee, a long-established body representing jointly the Ministry of Health and the Ontario Hospital Association. Projections of population growth were made by the HSRC to 2003; the choice of that year as the planning horizon was made by the ministry. Although this horizon was acknowledged to be short given the actual timelines applying to hospital construction and redevelopment, it was readily apparent that a later date would have resulted in significant errors arising out of imprecise projections based on the census data then available.

Application of these objective methodologies was regarded by many hospitals and their community representatives as a "numbers-driven" approach to decision-making on hospital capacity. It led to a number of criticisms, the most common being that the commission did not take sufficient account of local considerations, especially variations in the needs of the populations served and historical funding inequities.

Subsequent to the commission's final decisions and the release of its *Directions*, it was a rare hospital that did not complain that the methodology used had sized it with too few beds to meet the anticipated needs of the population it served. But in fact most hospitals were left with considerable flexibility in their approaches to the bed targets that had been set. This flexibility resulted from the HSRC's decision, taken after considerable debate on the issue, not to adjust observed admission/separation rates, the second of the two key variables used to determine bed capacity. The commission accepted each hospital's observed admission/separation rate as directly related to the needs of the community, district or region served, despite the fact that the rates varied widely throughout the province. The commission accepted these pre-existing rates as characteristic of local practice patterns and as reflecting possibly justifiable differences in the need for hospital-based services — or, at the least, as reflecting the perception of need by local physicians with admitting privileges. The HSRC did recognize, however, that this decision imposed an additional challenge and was somewhat unfair to those hospitals whose admission/separation rates were already low. With little or no ability to decrease this variable further, these hospitals had no choice but to reduce length of stay in order to meet the overall bed-capacity targets set by the commission. As it turned out, these hospitals were doubly disadvantaged. Between the release of the HSRC's *Directions* and its achieving its planning horizon in 2003, the resources provided to the hospitals from the ministry's hospital funding envelope proved inadequate to allow them to meet the commission's bed targets. As shown in table 1 and discussed later in this chapter, the carefully calculated acute-care-bed capacity in many communities has fallen short of what the commission predicted as necessary to meet the population's needs.

The issue of further categorizing patients in acute-care beds as those truly in need of this level of intensive care or those not in such need remained a bone of contention between the HSRC and the ministry for two years. To the commission it made great sense to differentiate between acute-care beds and those it referred to as subacute based on the relative need for care of patients in them. Such differentiation was essential to address the question of how many acute-care hospital beds were really needed, community by community. The commission defined subacute care as:

hospital-based in-patient care provided on a supervised in-patient unit of a hospital for individuals (patients) in need of slower paced recovery following surgery or short-term medical treatment and convalescence following an acute medical episode. The distinction between subacute and other types of care relates to the nature of the medical supervision, the degree of invasive diagnostics and procedures, the stability of the illness or disability, and the service requirements of the patient. Subacute care is aimed at patients who need to regain function and restore their independence prior to discharge to their home setting and reintegration into the community. Patients receiving subacute care are those who suffer from a loss of function as a result of an acute episode or extended stay in hospital, are deemed likely to regain function following a course of treatment and care focused on reactivation and restoration, and cannot receive conventional home-based services to manage their care requirements. (HSRC 1998b, 97)

The commission's intention in proposing this category of care (which has been adopted elsewhere and includes most patients categorized as ALC) was to identify the proportion of acute-care beds being filled by patients who did not need that level of care and to have the ministry fund those beds at a lower rate. From an operational perspective, aggregating such beds into designated subacute wards would facilitate, as with "step-down" units and the like, more efficient staffing and the provision of a more appropriate range of services than scattering them among acute-care beds filled by patients who require more intensive care. Also, patients accommodated on subacute wards would experience a smoother transition when discharged to their homes, with or without home care, or to long-term-care facilities. From a policy perspective, the commission deemed that the lower level of funding associated with subacute beds would serve as an additional incentive for hospitals to collaborate more closely with Community Care Access Centres to get their patients out of hospital quickly and placed in alternative care.

The ministry, however, did not accept the commission's recommendation that subacute care be established as a separate funding category. Its decision on this, made as late as January 1999 (well after the HSRC had issued *Directions* in many communities that had identified the proportion of acute and subacute beds

Table 1

COMPARISON OF ACUTE-CARE BEDS IN PLACE MARCH 31, 2003, WITH HSRC TARGETS FOR 2003, BY OHA REGION AND HSRC GROUPING

	Acute-care beds, March 31, 2001	Acute-care beds, March 31, 2003	HSRC target 2003[1]
HSRC groups in region 1			
North Bay	184	186	164
Sault Ste. Marie	213	214	190
Sudbury	395	381	420
Thunder Bay	314	314	368
Total	1,106	1,095	1,142
HSRC groups in region 2			
Brockville	103	103	103
Frontenac, Lennox & Addington	454	438	477
Haliburton, Kawartha, Pine Ridge	433	448	566
Hastings & Prince Edward Counties	209	227	266
Ottawa	1,538	1,318	1,341
Pembroke	97	93	104
Stormont, Dundas & Glengarry, Prescott & Russell Counties	147	136	157
Total	2,981	2,763	3,014
HSRC groups in Greater Toronto area (416 and 905 area hospitals from regions 3 and 4)			
Total	7,716	7,414	8,180
HSRC groups in region 4 (excluding 416 and 905 area hospitals)			
Brant	191	176	222
Hamilton-Wentworth	1,207	1,061	1,127
Niagara	761	647	754
Waterloo	553	575	597
Total	2,712	2,459	2,700
HSRC groups in region 5			
Essex	679	548	692
Kent	168	171	197
Lambton	184	182	240
London	946	898	1,081
Total	1,977	1,799	2,210
Grand total	16,492	15,530	17,246

Sources: Compiled by the Ontario Hospital Association from these sources: Daily Census, MOH-LTC; HSRC Bed and Place Chart; HSRC *Directives;* Discharge Abstract Database, MOH-LTC.
Note: All data exclude hospitals in any of the rural and northern networks.
[1] Includes acute beds, subacute beds and growth beds.
[2] Calculated as alternate level of care (ALC) patient days in 2002/03 divided by 365. Note that the reporting of the ALC portion of a patient's stay is inconsistent across hospitals and over time within individual hospitals. However, the overall provincial trend of the proportion of ALC patient days appears to be stable.

Beds over/ under target		Approximate ALC beds 2002/03[2]	March 31, 2003 acute-care beds less approx. ALC beds 2002/03	Approximate acute-care beds over/ under target after subtracting ALC beds	
N	%			N	%
22	13.4	43	143	-21	(12.8)
24	12.6	51	163	-27	(14.2)
-39	(9.3)	45	336	-84	(20.0)
-54	(14.7)	47	267	-101	(27.4)
-47	(4.1)	186	909	-233	(20.4)
0	–	16	87	-16	(15.5)
-39	(8.2)	68	370	-107	(22.4)
-118	(20.8)	28	420	-146	(25.8)
-39	(14.7)	27	200	-66	(24.8)
-23	(1.7)	177	1,141	-200	(14.9)
-11	(10.6)	4	89	-15	(14.4)
-21	(13.4)	23	113	-44	(28.0)
-251	(8.3)	343	2,420	-594	(19.7)
-766	(9.4)	684	6,730	-1,450	(17.7)
-46	(20.7)	4	172	-50	(22.5)
-66	(5.9)	79	982	-145	(12.9)
-107	(14.2)	88	559	-195	(25.9)
-22	(3.7)	85	490	-107	(17.9)
-241	(8.9)	256	2,203	-497	(18.4)
-144	(20.8)	26	522	-170	(24.6)
-26	(13.2)	11	160	-37	(18.8)
-58	(24.2)	9	173	-67	(27.9)
-183	(16.9)	50	848	-233	(21.6)
-411	(18.6)	96	1,703	-507	(22.9)
-1,716	(10.0)	1,565	13,965	(3,281)	(19.0)

in the hospitals concerned), was to continue to treat the sizing of subacute care as part of the hospital's complement of acute-care beds. Although the ministry gave no reason for this decision, the HSRC speculated that it wished to avoid opening a can of worms. If it had accepted the commission's analysis of the cost of subacute care and separated out the funding of those beds, the ministry would have faced enormous pressure to do a full costing of all aspects of acute care and the host of other activities engaged in by acute-care hospitals, the funding of which had for years been encompassed in global budgets. The commission thought it likely that the ministry just did not want to face what it knew would be a long and complex analytical process. Furthermore, neither the ministry nor the province's hospitals possessed the data necessary to engage in such a process, though a few hospitals participated in what was known as the Case Cost Group.[10] Incredible as it may seem from a business perspective, since the introduction of global budgeting nobody knows what it costs to carry out specific procedures in hospital (from appendectomies to stress tests), as the necessary accounting systems have long since been abandoned. It would have constituted a huge challenge to open the hospitals' global budgets without the data necessary to support even an informed argument about their adequacy or inadequacy in relation to real costs.[11]

DECISION-MAKING CRITERIA

Soon after the commission was formed, as early as its second meeting, its members debated the question of what goals or characteristics of the hospital sector it should try to preserve and enhance, what its principal criteria should be as it approached the concept of hospital restructuring and, indeed, the broader subject of fostering the creation of a genuine health-services system. Three criteria were quickly identified, and these became the HSRC's mantra — the fundamental principles that it applied to every decision.

The first criterion was that community *accessibility* to the services concerned, be they hospital beds or emergency rooms, had to be at least maintained and preferably enhanced. The second was that every decision had to lead to enhanced *quality* of the service offered; the probability of a positive outcome for patients and their families had to increase, whether due to a diagnostic or therapeutic procedure, surgery, clinic visit, admission to hospital — any contact between a user and a hospital or other health-service provider. The HSRC's third criterion was that its *Directions* and recommendations had to lead directly to greater *cost-effectiveness (affordability)*, enabling the institutions and organizations affected to produce more benefit to patients and the community with every dollar spent, principally by reducing the proportion of expenditures on administration and operations (for example, the hospital's plant).

These three criteria — preservation or enhancement of accessibility, quality and affordability — were supplemented by an informal but overarching test to which the commission attached great importance. This was the "man in the moon test," or the fundamental wisdom of a proposition[12] — "If you were to explain to the man in the moon what you are doing, would he say, 'That makes sense'?" Everything the commission said or did had to be readily understood by people uninitiated in the acronym-ridden jargon of hospitals and health care. Above all, its decisions had to make sense intuitively, even to those unfamiliar with the circumstances applying in the institutions and communities affected. The "man in the moon test" and the three criteria of accessibility, quality and affordability served both the HSRC and health care in Ontario well.

Although responsibility for the implementation of its decisions was not within its purview — that rested with the affected institutions and the Ministry of Health — the commission was concerned about the impact of hospital restructuring on nurses, other staff members and physicians. While the commission did not have the power to force changes on unionized labour, it saw a need for some general principles regarding the workers affected by its decision to close an institution, transfer programs from one hospital to another, or merge two or more hospitals. The question was whether the burden of restructuring — unemployment, at worst — would fall entirely on the staff of the hospital or hospitals to be closed or would be shared among the employees of all the affected hospitals in a given community. Similarly, would physicians with admitting privileges in a hospital scheduled for closure have the right to comparable privileges in the surviving hospital or hospitals?

At the outset there was concern, shared by the HSRC, about the possibility of massive layoffs as well as disruption of patient care as a result of hospital restructuring. No one doubted that reorganization would have enormous consequences for health professionals and all personnel, including managers. The commission viewed labour adjustment as an important consideration and realized that existing collective agreements and employment and appointment contracts were inadequate to address the new world of restructuring. A new way of dealing with change had to be developed. When the HSRC began its work of restructuring it was impossible to estimate the number of jobs that would be affected. Considerable variability among the communities was expected. The best strategy seemed to be for the parties concerned to address the problem *locally* with the least possible amount of prescription or intrusion by the commission. Accordingly, the HSRC's *Directions* in each community included the requirement that all parties develop a human resources plan. The agreements made early in the restructuring process in Windsor, London and Sarnia were available as models.[13] In many communities the HSRC appointed facilitators to help hospitals and employee groups develop plans. The facilitators brought the parties together to develop city-wide or region-wide plans for labour adjustment as well as plans to address issues specific to particular hospitals or other concerns.

As it did with governance (see chapter 3), the appointment of facilitators to assist with local labour-adjustment plans proved invaluable. Most of the groups involved in labour-adjustment issues agreed that the requirement of such plans was necessary to address the many issues and procedures involved. The assistance of facilitators from outside the community was always helpful and frequently essential. Many groups were affected, both unionized and nonunionized employees, and the various collective agreements set out often competing and inconsistent staff reassignment and layoff provisions. Without the facilitators, chaos and gross unfairness may well have resulted. The commission was concerned that increased uncertainty or the perception of unfair treatment would cause the premature departure of many employees from hospitals slated to close, seriously compromising patient care.

The negotiations were facilitated by an amendment made to the provincial labour law through the *Public Sector Labour Relations Transition Act, 1997*,[14] which provided processes to enable expeditious decision-making with regard to competing union rights in hospitals being restructured. Although organized labour was strongly opposed to the Act when it was introduced, it later became clear that the hospitals, as employers, were leery of the potential outcomes of the processes and tried to prevent the affected unions from triggering the Act's provisions.

As the commission's *Directions* began to appear and people realized the number of hospitals was going to be greatly reduced, the question of physicians' rights came to the fore at the Ontario Medical Association. This subject was raised at dinner meetings attended by the commission's Duncan Sinclair and Mark Rochon and the OMA president, William Orovan, a Hamilton-based urologist, and general secretary David Pattenden. Although it kept a close "watching brief" on the commission's work and many matters were discussed at those meetings, during the hospital-restructuring phase the OMA was not bothered save by this issue of securing hospital privileges elsewhere for physicians in hospitals facing closure or merger. In mid-1997 the HSRC appointed a task force[15] to identify issues arising out of its work, especially as they affected the medical staffs of the large academic centres in Toronto, London and Ottawa, and to recommend solutions. The task force came up with a number of guiding principles, including the following: the appointment process for medical staff should be open and fair; explicit criteria should be developed for the appointment, reappointment and evaluation of the medical staff, and for resource allocation relevant to working conditions (operating room time and the like); the appointments of physicians affected by restructuring should be maintained (through transfer to other hospitals); and the impact of hospital restructuring on patient care should be minimized.[16] These principles were embedded in the commission's *Notices* and *Directions* relating to Metropolitan Toronto, London and Ottawa, which served as templates for other communities. A few negative comments were received about a small number of hospitals that insisted on "home field advantage" and had not proceeded in a "fair and equitable" manner. But the OMA and physicians generally were satisfied with and served by the processes that the affected hospitals subsequently put in place.

What are the results of the commission's work? Today, five years after its "sunset," the scene is obviously transformed. From Thunder Bay (August 1996) through to the Niagara region, North Bay and Sault Ste. Marie (March 1999), a total of 22 communities, districts or regions were subject to binding *Directions* that reshaped the hospital landscape, primarily by reducing the number of buildings and organizations in order to establish fewer but larger hospitals. A total of 31 public hospitals were ordered to close and the minister was advised to close six private and six Provincial Psychiatric Hospital sites. Four hospitals were subsumed by the programs and activities of others. Other hospitals were amalgamated into entirely new, larger organizations. And 10 hospitals were ordered to form joint executive committees (JECs) to provide shared governance of previously separate organizations.

RESULTS

One of the criticisms most frequently directed at the commission, both upon the release of its *Directions* and subsequently, was that it did not provide hospitals with a sufficient number of acute-care beds to meet current and anticipated needs. This complaint has grown increasingly shrill as waiting for admission to hospital has become more prevalent and prolonged. The question of whether the commission underestimated the need for beds in Ontario's public hospitals in 2003 is addressed in table 1. The HSRC's targets were compared with the actual number of acute-care beds available by region and community in 2001 and 2003. To account for the fact that the total number of acute-care beds includes those the commission had recommended be reclassified as subacute, the number occupied by ALC patients[17] has also been subtracted, to arrive at the number really available to patients presenting with conditions that require an acute-care bed. The data demonstrate clearly that:

> The HSRC's targets for acute in-patient capacity have not been met in any community or region. When adjusted for accommodation of ALC patients, the total number of acute-care beds available in 2003 fell short of the *Directions* by 19 percent — a significant margin indeed. Nine percent of that shortfall can be attributed to continued occupation of those beds by (ALC) patients who would be more cheaply and, arguably, better cared for elsewhere, but fully 10 percent is a result of a lack of budgetary resources in 2003 to open and staff beds sufficient to meet the HSRC's targets.

> The shortfall varies greatly, from a low of 12.8 percent in North Bay, to over twice that in Thunder Bay and Lambton, to over 20 percent in many communities. But in no region does the number of available acute-care beds deviate far from the average of only 80 percent of the commission's carefully calculated predictions of need.

> Between 2001 and 2003 the gap between the total number of beds available and the HSRC's targets widened; the number of staffed acute-care beds shrank by nearly 6 percent!

It is impossible to say whether the HSRC's *Directions*, based on its predictions of acute-care needs in those communities in which it worked, were too generous, too parsimonious or just right. The simple fact is that they have not been met. The failure to differentiate subacute- from acute-care beds and the continued filling of the latter with ALC patients compounds the problem that, in 2003, Ontario's public hospitals contained only 80 percent of the acute-care capacity predicted as necessary by the HSRC. It is no wonder there are long waiting lists for admission to hospital!

HOSPITAL NETWORKS

In the course of the HSRC's study of public hospitals, particularly those in Ottawa and Metropolitan Toronto, it became apparent that something had to be done to coordinate the completely separate thrusts of many hospitals in five areas: women's health; children's health; rehabilitation; mental health and addictions; and, in Ottawa particularly, health services in the French language. A review of the spectrum of services and programs being offered showed that while many hospitals were involved and services were available to meet apparent needs, there was a public perception of these as "orphan" fields — disadvantaged in the struggle for recognition and resources in the face of "cutbacks." This problem was confounded by claims of "ownership" on the part of some — for example, children's health by Toronto's Hospital for Sick Children, women's health by Toronto's Women's College Hospital and French-language services by Ottawa's Montfort Hospital — claims vigorously resisted (and resented) by those with vested interests and proud records in the areas concerned. The commission considered the issues and developed a different approach in each of the five areas.

The formation of networks seemed the most sensible overall approach. In Ottawa, the commission ordered the newly consolidated Ottawa Hospital (including the Ottawa Heart Institute), the Children's Hospital of Eastern Ontario and the Sisters of Charity (offering complex continuing-care and nursing-home services) to become fully designated as bilingual under the requirements of the *French Language Services Act*. And it ordered the Montfort Hospital to lead the development of a network of hospitals in the city and region: the purpose of the French Language Services Network was to improve access of the francophone population to a complete spectrum of health services available in French.

In Metropolitan Toronto, the commission ordered the creation of the Addictions and Mental Health Foundation, drawing together into a single organization the Provincial Psychiatric Hospital, the Queen Street Mental Health Centre, the Addiction Research Foundation Clinical Institute, the Donwood Institute, the Mental Health and Addiction Services Corporation and the Clarke Institute of Psychiatry. The HSRC also recommended the formation of a single governance structure among all Metro Toronto hospital-based providers of mental health services to improve coordination among them and patient access to care. To facilitate coordination of rehabilitation services, the commission ordered the consolidated Toronto Rehabilitation Hospital to develop a network of the several specialty hospitals that provide rehabilitation services in the city. With respect to children's health, a task force representing the University Avenue Hospitals (University Health Network, Mount Sinai Hospital and the Hospital for Sick Children) was ordered to prioritize the configuration of obstetrical services in the neighbourhood. In addition, a Children's Health Network was established under the leadership of the Hospital for Sick Children, with a view to defining the standards necessary to provide babies and children with high-quality care at all levels ranging from routine to rare and to facilitate communication and co-ordination among all hospitals providing pediatric services in the city. After receiving unofficial approval from the ministry, the commission recommended the establishment of an agency for the support of women's health research, now known as the Ontario Women's Health Council and funded to the tune of $10 million annually. The council is charged with fostering studies throughout Ontario leading to the discovery of new and better ways of meeting women's needs for health services of all kinds.

RURAL AND NORTHERN HOSPITALS

In June 1988, by which time the commission was well along in its restructuring of urban hospitals, it extended its scope to include the much larger number of hospitals that serve Ontario's rural, northern and remote communities. The great majority of these are small institutions located some distance from one another, serving communities that are themselves small and often accessible only by road, making it difficult for patients to get to larger, referral hospitals, especially in winter. In most if not all of these communities, hospitals have difficulty recruiting and retaining the health professionals, especially specialist physicians, they need to offer even a modest range of programs in surgery, obstetrics and internal medicine.

From the outset it was obvious that the commission's approach to rural, northern and remote hospitals had to be very different from its approach to urban hospitals. Whereas the criterion of preserving or improving physical accessibility hardly applied in big cities with good transportation systems, it certainly did in Ontario's many small, rural and remote communities. There was never any thought of closing many, if any, of the small hospitals that are vital to people in widely distributed and isolated communities. In addition, the utilization benchmarks incorporated in the HSRC's methodologies were derived from best practices observed in urban hospitals; they were completely inappropriate for small hospitals where few patients present with like conditions.

The commission's approach was facilitated by the ministry's release of two documents bearing on small, northern and remote hospitals. The first of these set out a policy framework — guidelines to apply to hospitals, DHCs, community-based health-service providers and the ministry itself when planning for restructuring (Ontario Ministry of Health and Long-Term Care 1997). They called for the creation of health care networks to facilitate coordination of the work of all health-service providers in a particular community/district, first by linking together the hospitals in adjacent communities. Priority was to be given to ensuring the availability of services 24 hours a day. The second document contained a set of tools and a planning methodology to help DHCs, hospitals and other providers with the practical work of forming networks (Ontario Ministry of Health and Long-Term Care 1988).

This step by the ministry, pursued in collaboration with the Ontario Hospital Association, DHCs and the Registered Nurses Association of Ontario, came as a direct result of the HSRC's early work in Lambton County, where it had ordered the Charlotte Eleanor Englehart Hospital in Petrolia, a rural community, to establish a JEC with the Sarnia General Hospital and St. Joseph's Health Centre. The JEC's membership was to be drawn from the boards of the three hospitals. Its mandate was to oversee the provision of all hospital services and to consolidate, coordinate and streamline all administrative and related services under a common set of policy directions, clinical leadership and a single chief executive officer. Similar linkages were ordered for hospitals in Kent County and later Haliburton, Kawartha and Pine Ridge counties.

Well short of merging two or more organizations outright, JECs were conceived, as described in chapter 3, as a way of integrating the activities of previously separate hospitals while retaining their traditions, cultures and values. They were seen as an effective way for the governances of denominational and nondenominational hospitals to join forces in service to their communities without offence to either canon law or the religious sensibilities of their supporters. The concept of JECs was not new; a few had been in place for some years prior to the commission's establishment.[18] Made up of members from their boards of governors, JECs permitted the participating institutions to have their cake and eat it too; their boards retained their power over the big issues of governance but at the same time could delegate executive authority to the combined body on matters relating to joint endeavours. The commission knew that many boards would need time to establish a balance between retaining governance and delegating executive powers. But it anticipated that, over time, JECs would prove to be a viable way for the hospital partnership to preserve its connections to the founding institutions while providing its combined services to the population in a completely seamless way. Once established and given time to work out any teething problems, JECs would be hard to unwind; they would prevent a slide back to the status quo ante.

With the ministry's policy framework in hand, the HSRC began by identifying Ontario's rural, northern and remote hospitals. It met with some of their representatives and the DHCs involved to discuss grouping them into "clusters" based on geographical proximity and the transportation links among the communities in which they were located. The commission's analysis focused on the communities in which the patients of each hospital lived, where and how frequently they accessed local services, and which hospitals they were referred to for secondary and tertiary care. Each cluster, or network, contained at least one secondary referral hospital; for example, the North Bay General Hospital was the referral centre for what the commission called the Nipissing/Temiskaming Network, which also comprised four smaller hospitals, in Englehart, Mattawa, Sturgeon Falls and New Liskeard. The network concept was based on the idea that membership in it would lead to improved coordination and quality of services by virtue of common clinical standards and leadership. Other goals were information-sharing and common information systems, identification of better ways of meeting the needs of patients and their families throughout the district, collaborative development of common human resource policies, and a larger proportion of resources spent on patient care as a result of savings with regard to administrative and related services.

The commission had fully intended to follow its normal procedure and issue *Notices of Intentions to Issue Directions,* followed, after receiving feedback, by *Directions* to the hospitals concerned to form these networks. In April 1999, however, the government, nervous about negative political consequences in rural ridings in the face of the impending election, removed the commission's power to issue binding *Directions*. Therefore a total of 16 networks, encompassing 98 rural and northern hospitals, were recommended but not ordered by the HSRC.

These ranged in size from two hospitals[19] to a maximum of nine.[20] Although a few further attempts were made to form networks, and one cluster was formed in accordance with the HSRC's model[21] (subsequently "undone" in 2002), the ministry's and the commission's concept of networking small rural, northern and remote hospitals remains yet another good idea waiting to be implemented.

What is the outcome of the commission's work? Most noticeable, perhaps, is the rationalization of previously duplicated hospital programs and services in large cities. We have also seen the emergence of larger, multi-institutional organizations that allow for unified governance of previously separate hospitals. Excess bed capacity has been removed and then some: the pendulum has swung too far, as pendulums tend to do, and now there is a demonstrable deficiency of acute-care capacity. Too many ALC patients remain in acute-care beds, hindering further increases in capacity for patients in urgent need of acute care — patients who lie on gurneys in emergency departments waiting for a bed. Premier McGuinty's Liberals campaigned in the fall of 2003 on a promise to reopen some 1,300 acute-care beds. That would go some way toward closing the gap (3,000+), still obvious in 2005, between the number of acute-care beds the HSRC recommended be in operation at its planning horizon in 2003 and the number actually available. Yet, as a result of implementation of the reinvestment recommendations linked to the commission's *Directions*, the capacity of Ontario's communities, districts and regions to provide long-term and home care has greatly increased since 1996. Because of the lag between the commitment of resources and the completion of construction, most of the increases in long-term-care capacity have only recently come online. It is obvious that yet further expansion of community-based care is needed throughout Ontario, especially as the population ages.

There is much yet to do in restructuring Ontario's public hospitals and linking them with the many other elements necessary to create a genuine system of health care.

NOTES

1. Hôtel Dieu, founded in 1443 in Beaune, France, was the first hospital to provide refuge and medical care for people suffering the worst effects of the Hundred Years War. Now a museum, it functioned continuously as a hospital until 1971.
2. Subsequently the budget reduction (7 percent) scheduled for the third year, 1998-99, was rescinded.
3. District Health Councils were dispanded by the Government of Ontario in the spring of 2005.
4. The Thunder Bay DHC was part of the Northwestern Ontario DHC until DHCs were eliminated in early 2005.
5. The recommendations in this report represented the council's advice to the minister of health on the issue of hospital restructuring. The report *Final Advice of the MTDHC to the Minister of Health on the Hospital Restructuring Project* (November 1995), developed by the Metropolitan Toronto DHC, was released as a companion document to the final report.
6. For example, the starting point for review of mental health beds was based on a 1993 Ontario government policy document, *Putting People First*, that outlined a framework for the reform of the province's mental health system and proposed a target bed ratio of 30 psychiatric beds for every 100,000 people in the province by 2003 (60 percent of these beds classified as acute in-patient and 40 percent as longer-term mental health). When *Putting People First* was published, the provincial average stood at 58 beds/100,000 with considerable variation across the provincial planning regions. The HSRC based its assessment of bed requirements for chronic care on ratios derived from the *Chronic Care Role Study* (1993) and the planning ratios used to size the chronic care sector as part of the restructuring project in Windsor (11.4 beds/1,000 population [75+] as a benchmark for the whole population).
7. For details see HSRC (2000b, appendix C).
8. Case Mix Groups (CMGs) is a Canadian patient classification system used to group and describe types of in-patients discharged from acute-care hospitals. Modelled after the American Diagnosis Related Groups (DRGs), they were developed by the Canadian Institute for Health Information using four criteria: patient groups had to make good clinical sense; be based on routinely collected data; be manageable in number; and be statistically homogeneous with respect to length of hospital stay. Based on most-responsible diagnosis, the CMG grouper assigns each hospital abstract to one of 25 mutually exclusive Major Clinical Categories (MCCs). MCCs are based on body systems (e.g., diseases of the circulatory system, diseases of the respiratory system). Within each MCC, cases are classified as medical or surgical and CMGs are assigned accordingly. Cases within the same CMG are then assigned to typical or atypical categories. Typical cases represent the completion of a full course of treatment at a single hospital. Atypical cases denote one of four categories: deaths, sign-outs, transfers and long-stay outliers.
9. Measured by the number of distinct case types (Case Mix Groups 851, "other factors causing hospitalization" and 910 "diagnoses not generally hospitalized") that could be handled on an ambulatory basis or diverted to other providers in either the health or the social service system.
10. A select group of hospitals in which studies are being conducted to determine the cost of accommodating and treating patients with specific diagnoses.
11. In fact an increasing number of "hospital reviews" are being conducted, primarily as a result of increasing deficits, to identify the reasons for apparent discrepancies between a hospital's funding and the range and volume of services it provides.
12. Conceived by Dr. Larry Wilson, Duncan Sinclair's predecessor as dean of medicine at Queen's University.

13 Prior to the establishment of the commission, hospitals and unions in Windsor, London and Sarnia negotiated framework agreements based on DHC reports. These path-breaking agreements dealt with the relevant issues in hospital labour adjustment.
14 SO 1997, c. 21, Schedule B.
15 Including three physicians: Dr. John Atkinson (J. Atkinson Health Care Professionals) (chair), an anaesthetist from Ottawa; Dr. Ruth Wilson, a family physician from Kingston; and Dr. John Jarrell, an obstetrician and gynecologist from Calgary and chief medical officer for the Calgary Regional Health Authority.
16 Medical Human Resources Fact Finders report to the HSRC, January 1998.
17 Calculated from hospital census data reported to the Ontario Hospital Association.
18 In Kingston, for example, a JEC had been in place for some years to coordinate the activities of the Kingston General, Hotel Dieu and St. Mary's of the Lake (later Providence Continuing Care Centre), together with the Kingston Psychiatric Hospital, Frontenac, Lennox and Addington Home Care (later CCAC), and Queen's University, as participants in the Academic Health Sciences Centre of Southeastern Ontario.
19 Alliston/Newmarket Network: Stevenson Memorial Hospital, Alliston; and York County Hospital, Newmarket.
20 Northeast Network: Anson General Hospital, Iroquois Falls; Bingham Memorial Hospital, Matheson; Chapleau Health Services, Chapleau; Kirkland and District Hospital, Kirkland Lake; Lady Minto Hospital, Cochrane; Notre Dame General, Hearst; Sensenbrenner Hospital, Kapuskasking; Smooth Rock Falls General, Smooth Rock Falls; and Timmins and District Hospital, Timmins.
21 The Huron/Perth Network, encompassing: Alexandra Marine and General Hospital, Goderich; Clinton Public Hospital, Clinton; Listowel Memorial Hospital, Listowel; Seaforth Community Hospital, Seaforth; South Huron Hospital, Exeter; Stratford General Hospital, Stratford; St. Mary's Memorial Hospital, St. Mary's; and Wingham and District Hospital, Wingham.

CHAPTER 5

RECOMMENDATIONS LINKED TO HOSPITAL RESTRUCTURING: CONSTRAINTS ON POWER

The commission's power, although unprecedented, was not nearly as great as the hospital community, other providers and the general public were led to believe by the media and perhaps by the government itself. Although the legislation that gave the HSRC its mandate did not, as the Catholic Health Association and others complained, put limits on what it could do, the power to direct the restructuring of Ontario's public hospitals was circumscribed by the simple reality that any recommendation affecting those hospitals required the government to spend money. Most of the recommended spending was for community-based alternatives for patients who could not be safely discharged from hospital without continuing care. And the commission did not have — nor should it have had — the power to commit the government to spend taxpayers' money. In fact, the reality that only the government could spend money constituted a financial limit on the HSRC's power, a limit that could have easily been translated into a political one had the government been inclined to use it that way. In effect, the link between the HSRC's power to order hospital restructuring and the government's power to accept, modify or reject its recommendations on reinvesting in and/or restructuring everything else put the HSRC in the spotlight and left the government safely backstage where it could pull the strings, either allowing or preventing implementation of the recommendations and *Directions*. The Harris government pulled off a clever trick — retaining all the power while creating the illusion of relinquishing a substantial amount of it.

In extremis, of course, had the HSRC been too politically troublesome, either in the nature of its recommendations or in its advocacy for their acceptance and implementation, the government could have shut it down at any time.

But, given the commission's profile and the hype about its independence and the need for it to be at arm's length from the government, this would have carried its own political risk. So both the government and the commission had to weigh, from opposite sides of the scale, the risks associated with every potential reaction to its *Directions* and recommendations, including that of an accelerated "sunset."

Not all hospital restructuring entailed changes affecting capacity. The commission's power to order changes to the governance and management of hospitals was not constrained save by the enabling legislation's reasonable requirement that the HSRC act in "the public interest"; it also had to adhere to existing government policy and, of course, the laws of the land. An equally reasonable requirement was that in gathering information and making decisions, the commission, like government decision-makers and all manner of tribunals and administrative bodies, act fairly and give those affected by its decisions an opportunity to make their views known in advance. In the context in which the HSRC was operating, that meant it was obliged to give the hospitals affected an opportunity to make their views known; but it did not have to go further than that. The Catholic Health Association had it partially right. Given the importance of the composition, structure, and quality of governance and management of hospitals, the commission did possess significant independent power to make changes that would be most unwelcome to those affected. But since the commission's mandate in phase I was to "rationalize" the province's public hospitals, the great majority of its actions, whether expressed as *Directions* or as *Recommendations*, entailed the spending of public money. It is fair to say that the majority of its decisions remained entirely in the hands of the government, primarily in those of the premier as advised by the Management Board of Cabinet and the minister of health.

The greatest impact was that associated with what the HSRC termed "reinvestment." This term was based partly on the premise that anticipated savings derived from hospital downsizing and consolidation would be reinvested elsewhere in health care — recall the government's commitment at the outset not to cut overall public spending on health care throughout the four years of its mandate. Furthermore, the commission was not restricted or constrained by any limit (except reasonableness, internally defined) when recommending the amount of reinvestment it thought necessary to meet the needs of the population for any health service. But, in general, the intention was to transfer funds out of the hospital envelope to finance the capital construction and operation of long-term-care beds and expansion of the rehabilitation and home-care services needed to accommodate alternative level of care (ALC) patients discharged from hospital into these community-based alternatives. The logic was compelling — substitute equally good or better care for much more costly hospital beds. The problem for the government, however, was that while increasing the capacity of home care was, in principle, fairly straightforward — it required only a transfer of resources from hospitals to Community Care Access Centres (CCACs) — the creation of more long-term-care beds was not so simple. The construction of new buildings would take some time and a lot of money up front; in the meantime the expense of keeping patients in high-cost hospital beds would continue. Bridge financing for three to four years was required at a time when the government was preoccupied with delivering on its campaign promise to reduce the provincial debt.

But expanding the capacity of community care was not the only problem with implications for the provincial cash flow. Closing hospitals also involved decommissioning costs. More significantly, consolidating hospital activities in fewer buildings required the government to open the provincial purse, to deal, for example, with human resource adjustment costs and fund the capital construction necessary to expand the emergency room or operating theatre or critical-care capacity of a single hospital ordered by the HSRC to provide a service that had previously been provided by two or more hospitals in the same community.

This created a monster problem. Classically, governments provide hospitals with "global budgets." In fact, these support only their annual operating costs (including depreciation of equipment); the capital requirements of renewing their buildings and infrastructure are considered primarily on a project-by-project basis. Typically, more capital projects are approved when governments are flush than in lean times. For the several lean years prior to the late 1990s, hospitals in Ontario had been starved for funds to maintain and renew their capital — buildings and building systems (heating, air-conditioning, etc.). They were used to protracted and difficult negotiations with the ministry over the capital projects they proposed, negotiations that usually yielded sums barely adequate to meet even their basic needs, much less their ambitions, even when supplemented by funds raised locally by capital campaigns.

The commission engaged architectural consultants[1] to help it estimate the costs of implementing recommendations related to the capital construction required to achieve restructuring (and ultimately to save operating costs). It should be noted that the HSRC examined and made recommendations related *only* to the capital construction needed for restructuring — to accommodate more patients from another hospital it had ordered to close or to cease offering those programs. The commission's failure to address the larger issue of what it would cost to bring aging buildings up to snuff (and up to modern building and fire codes) and to recommend that the government fund them was a source of great frustration to the hospitals and communities concerned. Predictably, in every instance, once the HSRC recommended cracking open the public purse, the hospitals built their cases for more money, more space and more extensive renewal of their infrastructure — the maximum they thought they could get out of the negotiation process. That process, of course, had the commission as a mere observer on the sidelines — an informed observer to be sure, but an observer nonetheless. Political and every other kind of influence remained very much part of the games played by insistent hospitals and their community representatives on one side and a harassed ministry with a huge and growing list of capital demands on the other. The ministry itself was caught between the imperative of getting on with implementing the HSRC's *Directions* and a management board extremely reluctant to spend money up front even against the commission's assurances of a dividend in the form of decreased operating costs down the road. To be fair, the management board was right to be cautious. Given that the government had already announced a sharp reduction in their global budgets (18 percent plus inflation between 1996-97 and 1998-99), most of the anticipated "savings" had already been squeezed out of hospitals one way or another by the time the HSRC issued its *Directions* and *Recommendations*.

During the first two years or so, the conflict between the government's determination to reduce spending as much and as rapidly as possible and the fact that implementation of the commission's *Directions* and *Recommendations* required the spending of money resulted in frustration on all sides; there was growing disenchantment with restructuring as a useful exercise. The HSRC and its members became increasingly frustrated, irritated and angry, first with the government's foot-dragging, even with respect to commenting on its *Recommendations,* and later with its obvious unwillingness to buy the argument that money had to be spent in the short term, particularly in support of capital construction and to beef up the capacity of home care to support hospital restructuring. In a letter to the minister of health in November 1997, covering its quarterly report, the chair wrote:

> The commission is concerned about…the continued and growing delay between our having issued recommendations on capital investment and operating reinvestments in home care,

long-term care, and subacute care in communities where final *Directions* have been issued. There is nothing more threatening to the work we have done, and are doing in hospital restructuring, than a real or apparent "disconnect" between the "book ends" of our *Directions* on hospital restructuring and the ministry's announcements of action on our recommendations on capital and, particularly, reinvestments in operating funding for community-based services. (Sinclair 1997)

He wrote again following a meeting in January 1998, almost two years after the commission had first met, saying, "One member went so far as to suggest that the commission consider 'downing tools' and put a 'hoist' on (further work) pending the announcement of decisions on our recommendations" (Sinclair 1998).

The urban hospitals affected to that point by the commission's work, many of which had by then bought into the basic idea of restructuring, became increasingly frustrated, while the long-term-care sector, perceiving itself both a major beneficiary of the reinvestment of money from the hospital envelope and the recipient of a lot more responsibility for the care of discharged patients, was beside itself with uncertainty. It was an increasingly tense time that did not end until the government's announcement, made jointly by Premier Mike Harris and health minister Elizabeth Witmer on April 28, 1998, of a significant reinvestment in home care and facility-based long-term care. Behind that announcement, of course, was analysis by the treasurer showing that Ontario's economic recovery had picked up steam and was on track for further growth. Forecasts of the increased revenue streams showed that modestly increased capital and some operational spending would not threaten steady reduction of the deficit. Another factor was that by the spring of 1998 the government was thinking about its re-election and the likely effects of continued stalling on hospital restructuring versus some good news about building new long-term-care facilities.

Ontario's downsizing of in-patient capacity in its psychiatric hospitals in the early 1970s remained in the public memory a vivid example of what not to do. In those days, research, the availability of safer and more effective pharmaceutical agents, and experience in other jurisdictions provided convincing evidence that a large proportion of patients with mental health problems who had been confined in hospital for long periods could be cared for safely and well as outpatients. The experience of living in community settings would also, for the great majority, result in marked improvement in both their underlying mental conditions and their quality of life. Accordingly, many were discharged from the sheltered and restricted environment of psychiatric hospitals. But funding and subsidized housing were inadequate. Insufficient amounts of planning and time were devoted to easing the transition to community living by assisting patients in the search for accommodation or training them to look after themselves in a challenging and stressful world. The transition was far too abrupt. Almost instantly many of the discharged patients became glaringly disadvantaged street people. Responsibility for their welfare fell directly and precipitously on municipal governments unprepared to meet it. It was several years before a community-based support structure evolved to provide them with the counsel and direct assistance with the challenges of daily living that should have been put in place before the first of them were discharged. The commission was determined to avoid creating a comparable situation for ALC patients in Ontario's acute-care hospitals. It made it as clear as words permit that no action should even be contemplated to downsize those hospitals unless and until the corresponding capacity was in place in long-term-care facilities and home care in each concerned community and region.

The obvious question, then, was: What constitutes corresponding capacity and how should it be distributed among the several providers of community-based care in the different regions of the province?

COMMUNITY CARE CAPACITY

It had become clear early in phase I that one of the principal challenges facing the commission was to find or develop planning measures and guidelines for community-based care, particularly long-term and home care — measures and guidelines that could be used to assess their capacity and competency to meet the needs of ALC patients. In fact, the absence of planning standards for long-term and home care was part of a larger problem that extended to facilities and community-based organizations adapted to provide services to patients with mental health disorders, to a lesser degree those requiring rehabilitation — all of whom were classified in the ALC category — or those then accommodated in acute-care hospital beds who would live permanently with severe disabilities. Accordingly, the HSRC set out soon after its formation to develop guidelines that would serve as a framework for rebalancing the provision of health services among hospitals, home care, long-term care, mental health care, rehabilitation and other forms of post-acute care, including in-patient subacute care.

The HSRC realized early on that one of the greatest challenges in its task of restructuring hospitals would be to fill quickly a huge policy void related to the issue of system-wide planning of health services. Part of the problem was a lack of information about current patterns of service utilization outside the hospital sector. Moreover, the situation was complicated by the absence of ministerial planning guidelines. The commission faced the daunting task of developing from the ground up a policy framework built inescapably on the imprecise foundation of wide variation in the utilization of long-term care, home care, supportive housing and other services across the province. The resultant guidelines, when applied, would have to produce relatively precise answers to such questions as: How much accommodation/service capacity must be created, where, at what cost, and who should pay, how much and what for?

The ultimate goal of this time-consuming and frustrating exercise was to put in place objectively derived planning standards that would relate the capacity required in each modality providing care to the population of the community, district or region to be served. Two years after its formation, the commission published the necessary guidelines (HSRC 1998a). They were the product of diligent work by the HSRC's staff and independent consultants as well as extensive consultations with all concerned service providers. The results were admittedly in the category of "the best that could be done" given the lack of data on the care of people by institutions and organizations providing community-based services. Many individuals and organizations commended the HSRC for taking up the challenge of developing explicit planning methodologies/ guidelines to equip the nonacute service sector to play its part in restructuring the health-services system. In a 1998 letter, the Faculty of Medicine at the University of Toronto wrote: "With the restructuring of the acute care hospitals and the appropriate use of acute care hospitals for the seriously ill only, increasingly students will receive clinical training in ambulatory settings and in the institutions covered by the 'rebuilding paper.' We therefore are pleased that the commission has recognized the importance of these sectors."

When developing this planning framework the commission quickly discovered that whereas the data available to support hospital restructuring were poor to barely adequate, those relating to other modalities of care were from grossly inadequate to nonexistent. Unlike the public hospitals that for years had contributed data to the Canadian Institute for Health Information in accordance with standards it developed, no such coordinating force existed for organizations providing home, long-term, mental health or rehabilitation care. Where records were kept, most were sketchy and their formats idiosyncratic to the organizations concerned. Few centralized databases existed at the time; those that did could not be readily correlated with databases originating in hospital-based care.

Although efforts are now being made to correct such deficiencies, in 1996 few data standards applied to out-of-hospital care, even to how recipients of care were identified. There was no possibility of reliably aggregating information on people transferred from one form of care to another — for example, a postoperative patient with a hip replacement receiving physical or occupational therapy first in a rehabilitation hospital, then in a long-term-care facility and finally at home with the assistance of home care. The commission did undertake a home-care project in which different data sets were linked. All patients who received home care within 30 days of their in-patient stay or procedure were classified as home-care recipients. The home-care utilization rates were determined for each Major Clinical Category (MCC) and for each Day Procedure Group (DPG), linking CIHI data[2] with services and registration files for each of the province's 38 home-care programs. This led to a ranking of home-care programs based on utilization rates and to the HSRC's adoption of the 25th percentile as its benchmark for the recommendation of reinvestments in underserved areas. Since 1996, when the commission first discovered the seriousness of this lack of information, some improvement has been made, but there is a long way to go.[3]

Mental Health Care

Forcing the development of rational standards on which to base its recommendations for community reinvestment were decisions relating to Thunder Bay, the first community in which the HSRC worked. There, the commission undertook to rationalize what had been the city's five, then four, hospitals — Thunder Bay Regional (previously Fort William's McKellar General and the Port Arthur General), St. Joseph's General, the Hogarth-Westmount (the result of a previous amalgamation of two chronic-care hospitals) and Lakehead Psychiatric. Deciding what to do about the latter brought to the fore an unanswerable question: What is the most appropriate balance between a hospital's in-patient capacity for psychiatric patients and the capacity of the community and region to care for them as outpatients?

Compounding the problem of setting guidelines for the capacity of community-based mental health services is the overlap and boundary between health services and social services. The distinction is hard to draw in any case but particularly for people with mental health problems living and being cared for in noninstitutional community settings. To complicate matters further, the services fall under the jurisdictions of two large ministries, the Ministry of Health and the Ministry of Community and Social Services. They operate in a very different style; in the health ministry most decision-making takes place at the centre, whereas "Com-Soc" leaves much more discretion and authority to its regional offices.

Focusing first on mental health services and hospital-bed capacity, the HSRC based its decisions on the results of two studies by the Ministry of Health that had established a target of 30 beds per 100,000 population as the appropriate guideline on which to base in-patient capacity (Ontario Ministry of Health 1994)[4]; the ministry later determined that 18 of those beds should be designated for patients with acute mental health problems and 12 for those requiring longer-term care (Ontario Ministry of Health 1995). Following its release of *Notices* advising the hospitals in Thunder Bay of its intention to order that those standards be met by 1999, the commission received a flood of expressions of concern from around the province that this target was too aggressive — there was insufficient time for the development of alternative support capacity in the community. After its subsequent analysis of the use of beds in all hospitals province-wide by mental health patients (HSRC 1998a, 49-60), the HSRC reaffirmed its support for the guideline of 30 beds/100,000 as appropriate in the long term but modified the pace of its application. It adopted two interim guidelines — 37 beds/100,000 (21 acute and 16 long-term) by the year 2000 and 35 beds/100,000 (21 acute and 14 long-term) by 2003. Two key questions remained: How should community-based services for mental health patients be restructured? How much organizational capacity and money are required both in the interim and at steady state? After consulting with experts and holding prolonged, in-depth discussions with a wide variety of stakeholders, the commission reached three conclusions:

> Given Ontario's diversity and the needs of its population for mental health (and related social) services, those questions would be best answered on a regional basis.

> Only people on the ground with knowledge and experience of the needs of their region and their community-by-community capacities to develop and provide good care for patients and families burdened with illnesses of this kind could answer the questions effectively.

> Although the commission was resolutely opposed to the principle of "directed" funding, it agreed that an exception should be made to protect

an expanded regional mental health funding envelope. It recommended that this be put in the hands of regional Mental Health Agencies (MHAs) charged with implementing the interim guidelines and meeting the ministry's goal in *Putting People First* of having community care claim 60 percent of the mental health budget and 40 percent of the institutional-care budget by 2003. The MHAs were to decide where the proportion of funds going to community care would be spent to meet best the needs of people living with mental illness in the communities throughout their regions.

Accordingly, in its first quarterly report to the minister of health in June 1996 the commission gave notice of its intention to recommend the establishment of regional MHAs to protect the mental health envelope from being diverted to other purposes and to act as "purchasing agents" for a spectrum of mental health services, both hospital- and community-based. Although it subsequently developed specific guidelines based on its analysis of Ontario-wide needs for various categories of in-patient mental health care (acute, long-term, child/adolescent, forensic), it recognized that it did not have, and would be unable to get within the time available, the data necessary to do much more. Accordingly it shunted to the Ministry of Health responsibility for developing provincial standards, benchmarks and guidelines for the provision of community-based mental health services, including vocational rehabilitation, crisis intervention, housing supports, case management, the "domhostel" and related services of the Ministry of Community and Social Services, and other support services. The HSRC conceived regional MHAs as time-limited but powerful catalysts for change within their regions, guideline/benchmark development by the ministries concerned, and rapid improvement in the care of people with mental illness. Its goal was to promote development of provincial policies/guidelines to ensure the sharing of best practices among the various regions and the availability of a comprehensive range of mental health services in all regions of the province.

The Ministry of Health initially supported the concept of MHAs but later changed its tune, due, at least in part, to vigorous lobbying by the government's professional psychiatric staff. The public-sector unions representing the psychiatrists and other workers in the Provincial Psychiatric Hospital (PPH) system did not embrace the MHA concept, except by the neck to strangle it. They saw that the establishment of these agencies would dilute their leverage in central bargaining regarding wages and workloads. The government dragged its feet interminably on this recommendation, perhaps because it viewed MHAs as the thin edge of the wedge of generalized devolution/regionalization, to which succeeding Ontario governments were opposed; or perhaps because the establishment of MHAs would rock the boat too vigorously. In any case silence reigned, despite what the commission perceived as strong support from the communities and regions affected for the concept of giving MHAs the authority to manage the transition to a better balance of institutional and community-based mental health services.

In 1999, concerned after two years and more about the lack of progress and keenly aware of an urgent need for a community-based process to support the implementation of restructuring mental health beds, the HSRC submitted to the minister a separate policy document. Titled *Advice to the Minister of Health on Building a Community Mental Health System in Ontario,* it recommended that:

> the minister of health establish nine Mental Health Implementation Task Forces (MHITFs) throughout the province, to remain in place only until PPH restructuring was completed[5]

> MHITFs be vested with responsibility for overseeing PPH restructuring and for making recommendations to the Ministry of Health regarding the allocation of transitional funds (available to implement restructuring), as well as the reallocation of funds as a result of PPH restructuring

Finally realizing that something had to be done, the government accepted the HSRC's recommendation that mental health reform be led by district/regional groups close to the communities affected. It began to establish task forces as conduits for the development of local/regional plans of action. A total of nine were established in 2000 and 2001, mandated to recommend local and regional improvements to mental health services across the province.[6] The government's task forces, however, were a mere shadow of the MHAs originally proposed by the HSRC; they controlled no budgets and had no catalytic power to accelerate the development of guidelines/benchmarks for population-based allocation of resources to mental health services in the community. Such guidelines remain to this day on the distant horizon. The reports of the task forces, submitted in 2003, are still "under consideration" (Ontario Ministry of Health and Long-Term Care 2002).

Home Care

Home care is also an admixture of what most people think of as health and social services, health services being those required to treat people who are ill or injured, and social services being those required by people who need help with the functions of daily living — bathing, cleaning, shopping, meal preparation and the like. The commission's analysis of reported home-care caseloads over the three years ending in 1995-96 indicated that approximately 30 percent of the care involved the provision of social services (community-referral home care); the remainder involved the provision of health services to clients who presented with two different kinds of need: for short-term care, most after discharge from hospital pending a return to independent living; and for home care over the long term, sometimes on a continuing basis.

Given its need to determine initially how well home care could substitute for hospital care, the HSRC concentrated first on short-term, or what it called postacute home care.[7] Nearly half (46 percent) of all home-care services then provided in Ontario were in this category — initiated in patients' homes within 30 days of discharge from a hospital bed or after same-day surgery and continuing for variable periods up to one year. The remainder, involving about one-quarter of home-care clients, including those discharged subsequently to a long-term-care facility and who received home care for more than 180 days, were considered in a parallel study to determine the community's capacity for long-term home care. Although the definitions were necessarily applied strictly for the purpose of developing population-based guidelines, the commission was well aware that many patients/clients fall into more than one category. The distinctions between acute and long-term health services and between health and social services are artificial and therefore distressingly arbitrary.

As with community-based mental health services, the data on home care were sketchy at best. In the CCACs — the organizations responsible for the provision of home care in Ontario — record-keeping and data-management technology and personnel were both rudimentary and sparse. Also, the ministry and the CCACs themselves had paid little attention to developing the ability to connect information on home-care services with that relating to the care of clients previously in hospital or subsequently in long-term-care facilities. Here, too, a silo of care was barely connected with other, closely related silos. The result was huge cost to two important concepts: continuity of care for patients/clients transferred from one service provider to another, and the operation of a genuine system of health care.

Examining the data available, the commission discovered a disturbing three-and-a-half-fold variation in utilization rates among Ontario's 38 community/regions-based home-care programs and roughly corresponding differences in funding. Having recognized the glaring funding disparities, the ministry had adopted the policy that any new money available for home care should go to the programs deemed to be underfunded; the goal was to improve equity in relation to the age- and gender-adjusted demographic profile of the population served.

The HSRC took a more analytical approach. It tried to determine the underlying reasons for the large intercommunity/regional differences in service capacity. Using hospital and census data, it estimated the number of hospitalizations among the community/regional population served in 1995-96 for each MCC and Day-Procedure Group (DPG), and applied as a benchmark the 75th percentile (as it had for length of hospital stay) across the range of observed home-care utilization rates for each category and group. This allowed for the calculation of a population-based target in each of the 38 programs. This approach revealed that the variability in capacity was attributable not to comparable variability in the need for home care, but to the effectiveness of different community/regional CCACs in advocating, entirely legitimately, for more money to meet the needs of their populations. It also provided underpinning for the commission's calculation that by 2003 home care in Ontario would have to serve nearly a quarter of a million postacute clients, those newly discharged from hospital or from day surgery — a ratio of 2,025 postacute home-care cases per 100,000 population. This represented an increase in capacity of nearly 50 percent over the average number of postacute home-care episodes observed in Ontario in the three years 1993-94 to 1995-96.

The HSRC then applied an algorithm to convert that target into the funding necessary to achieve it, taking into account the differing service intensity and cost of caring for patients in each MCC and DPG and factoring in case management, equipment and travel costs. It recommended a 23 percent increase in provincial expenditures in support of postacute home care by 2003, a total of $165 million in 1998, to be distributed based on the distribution of hospital populations rather than on regional geography. It also recommended that discussions be initiated immediately between the Ministry of Health and CCACs in order to develop a province-wide information system to support both planning for further development of home-care services and an accountability framework to assess the benefits accruing to clients/patients against the money spent.

Many arguments remain about the efficacy of home care. Its proponents believe that home care can substitute for a significant proportion of the acute rehabilitation and complex continuing care now provided in hospitals and also offer qualitative and financial benefits. One qualitative benefit is the strong preference of most patients to be cared for at home rather than face isolation in a hospital, away from their families. While some contend that home care supports family caregivers, others believe that it shifts a greater burden of both cost and care onto the family. Much of the limited research on home care available to the commission in 1996-97 did not support the underlying assumptions regarding its effectiveness (including cost-effectiveness) as a substitute for institutionally based care (Weissert 1992; Welch, Wennberg and Welch 1996). However, it has also been shown that, with coordinated discharge planning, home care following hospitalization is of greater benefit to the patient and costs less than similar care provided in hospital (Saskatchewan Health Services Utilization and Research Commission 1998). Despite the lack of conclusive evidence, the commission accepted the conventional wisdom that home care is a necessary and will be an increasingly important player in the modern health care system that the HSRC was charged with fostering.

More recently, however, a consensus seems to have emerged on the importance of home care as a substitute for services provided in an acute-care facility (Hollander and Chappell 2002; Coyte and McKeever 2001). The Standing Senate Committee on Social Affairs, Science and Technology and the Romanow Commission have both advocated expanding home care, particularly short-term acute care. To quote the latter:

> Because home care has become a partial substitute for care that was previously provided primarily in hospitals or by physicians, and because of the value of effective home care services both to individuals and the health care system, a strong case can be made for taking the first step in 35 years to expand coverage under the Canada Health Act…The commission recommends that the definition of what is covered under the CHA should immediately be expanded to include medically necessary home care as well as diagnostic services…Because of the significant costs that would be involved in including all home care services under the CHA, priorities should be placed on the most pressing needs… These three areas — mental health, post-acute care, and palliative care — should be the first three home care services to be included under a revised CHA. (Royal Commission on the Future of Health Care in Canada 2002)

The *First Ministers' Accord on Health Care Renewal* of 2003 also cites the need to "improve access to a basket of services in the home and community to improve the quality of life of many Canadians by allowing them to stay in their home or recover at home."[8]

Long-Term Care

Closely related to its development of capacity and reinvestment guidelines for home care was the commission's study of the long-term-care sector in all its diversity — hospitals of different types with long-term-stay beds, nursing homes, homes for the aged, supportive housing, long-term home care, attendant care and adult day care. As with mental health care, home care and other health services that are offered in the community rather than in institutions, the primary question was a definitional one: What proportion of recipients would be best served by the different levels and types of care available? A confident answer required analysis of health records to ascertain the needs of those people for health as opposed to social services. For those needing health services, the HSRC had to distinguish between people requiring short-term care and those requiring long-term care. Then it had to determine, for both groups, the appropriate level of intensity and technological sophistication of care necessary to help patients deal with their particular illness or disability. Here again, the commission was blocked by both a lack of data and the incompatibility of such record systems as were available among the several providers of long-term care.

There were also profound differences among providers in their approaches to care. Home care, for example, refers to its recipients as *clients*, studiously avoiding the term *patients*, which is common in hospitals and among providers of health services generally. Those in long-term-care facilities are generally referred to as *residents*, a term suggesting even more decision-making autonomy than *clients* and a great deal more than the implied dependency of *patients*.

The commission started with a question: Where are people receiving long-term-care services now? An analysis of the long-term-care sector in 1995-96 revealed that slightly over 22 percent of all Ontario residents aged 75 or over were receiving some form of long-term care. Although their distribution among the six major contributors to publicly subsidized long-term care varied from region to region, on average, province-wide, the majority (over 45 percent) lived in long-term-care facilities (nursing homes or homes for the aged). Somewhat fewer but still a large proportion (37 percent) lived at home supported by long-term home-care services. In addition to these big programs, 7 percent of people 75 or over lived in supportive housing; 3.5 percent lived at home and received, rather than home care, attendant and adult day care supplied by community support programs through the social services ministry. Of the remainder, 6.5 percent were in what were then called chronic care (now known as complex continuing care) hospitals, and 1 percent occupied ALC beds in the province's acute-care hospitals.

The province-wide distribution was, however, as with home-care services, far from even. As illustrated in table 2, an assessment[9] of the 1995-96 utilization of long-term care in each county/region and for the province revealed a range of 175 places[10] per 1,000 people (75 years of age or over) in some counties and regions to over 400 in others. There was comparable variability among the six types of long-term care. It quickly became apparent to the commission that in all communities and regions the placement decisions of CCACs rested more on the availability of beds and places than on a match between the care that was available and the specific needs of the person. This is the result to be expected when the needs of the population exceed the capacity to meet them.

A compounding factor was the ongoing disagreement, primarily between the hospital and long-term-care sectors, on the best means of assessing the relative care needs of their patients/clients/residents — their degree of dependency on others to provide both health care and help with the requirements of daily living. The hospital sector had accepted the relatively new Minimum Data Set[11] as the most appropriate system for categorizing its patients' needs for continuing care, simple or complex, and identifying their level of dependence. By 1997, however, this tool had been used to assess the needs of continuing-care patients only in Metropolitan Toronto, the Niagara Region and Thunder Bay. An alternative, the Alberta classification system,[12] basically a funding tool on which the Ministry of Health depended, had been in use for several years in long-term-care facilities. The hospitals maintained that the Alberta system had limited applicability to health care or health-system planning. Those representing nursing homes and homes for the aged agreed that while the MDS/RUGS III assessment tool was more widely applicable than the Alberta system, it was much more expensive to implement and apply repeatedly to their residents (whose needs often changed rapidly and dramatically as they aged) than to hospital patients (whose numbers were much smaller and whose conditions were more stable). Rather than mediate or arbitrate this disagreement, the ministry sat on the fence and avoided making a decision on which assessment system to adopt both for the purpose of funding and the far more important purpose of matching people with the type and amount of long-term care most appropriate to their needs.

Given the urgent need for some credible guidelines to accompany its recommendations on reinvestment in long-term care, the commission was forced to

Table 2

UTILIZATION OF LONG-TERM-CARE SERVICES BY PERSONS AGED 75 AND OVER

LTC modality	Utilization of LTC per 1,000[1]		
	Minimum	Maximum	Provincial average
Alternate level of care beds	0.0	7.2	2.3
Chronic beds	2.9	26.4	14.1
Nursing homes/homes for the aged beds	57.4	176.5	100.7
Supportive housing	0.0	57.1	15.2
Home care	39.4	157.5	81.9
Community support services	0.0	34.2	7.8
Total LTC	174.5	402.7	221.9

Source: HSRC (1997b).
[1] Long-term-care beds or equivalent places per 1,000 people over the age of 75.

take a number of shortcuts. Beginning with hospitalized patients and extrapolating from the available MDS/RUGS III data (which categorize continuing-care patients based on dependence and care requirements according to seven levels of care,[13] three of which[14] can be provided only by hospitals), the HSRC developed the guideline of approximately 6.5 beds needed per 1,000 people aged 75 or over. After inviting and receiving feedback from the community and the providers affected, it increased the figure to 8.23 beds per 1,000, with the stipulation that it include respite care and palliative care in addition to complex continuing care.[15]

To make clear the intended function of what had previously been referred to as chronic care hospitals, and to distinguish these from acute-care hospitals, the commission adopted the practice of referring to hospitals that provided care to long-term patients as complex continuing care hospitals.

With respect to the distribution of residents in nursing homes and homes for the aged, in the absence of the capacity to generate more credible and useful data the commission reluctantly decided to accept the currently observed rates of utilization of long-term care among the different providers as a surrogate or proxy for the real needs of the population. The commission was aware that gradually, over many years, these homes had been transformed by their accommodation of increasingly elderly residents with debilitating health problems that restricted their ability to carry out the activities of daily living. They had changed from primarily residential facilities — institutional homes, in fact — to true nursing homes for people highly dependent on health and support services in addition to accommodation, meals, laundry, entertainment and other residential services. It was also aware of the increasingly alarmed complaints from the long-term-care sector that its funding did not permit the levels of staffing and expertise necessary to provide residents with the intensity of health services they required. The commission realized that if an assessment method or tool like MDS/RUGS III were to be applied to all long-term-care patients in hospital, clients of home care, and residents of long-term-care facilities and supportive housing, the results could well show that many people were being accommodated by facilities incapable of providing the services they needed; conversely, they could well show that people were being accommodated by facilities capable of providing services far more extensive and sophisticated than required for their degree of illness or disability. But under the imperative to develop guidelines quickly on which to base its reinvestment recommendations, and lacking the evidence necessary to do otherwise, the commission used the current rates of utilization as a surrogate for the number of long-term-care beds required in each community and region.

In contrast to its approach to guidelines for length of hospital stay and for acute-home-care capacity, where it targeted the 75th percentile of the observed range, the commission picked the 25th percentile of the sum of long-term-care and qualified ALC patients in hospital together with those currently in long-term-care beds as the target for the aggregate long-term-care capacity in each community or region. It chose the bottom rather than the top quartile because it believed strongly, based on extensive consultations, that, as an overarching principle, the government's reinvestment in supportive housing and comparable home-based community care should take priority over facility-based care. After calculating against the 25th percentile of observed utilization the number of long-term-care placements required for 12 age/gender groupings ranging from 0 to 14 years to 85 years and older, it applied population-growth estimates to 2003 for each community and region. Given the wide variation in utilization, and accepting the conventional wisdom (and the ministry's policy direction) that they reflect different needs, the HSRC divided northern and southern Ontario into separate groupings for planning purposes; more generous targets were applied to northern communities and regions. The results were dramatic. Whereas in 1996 only 7 communities/regions across the province had fewer long-term-care beds and places than required (a total deficiency of only 3,337 beds/places), by 2003 there would be 22 out of 38 regions requiring additional beds/places — a five-fold increase, taking population growth and aging into account.

After receiving feedback on its application of the proposed guidelines, the commission changed its target upward to the average (50th) rather than the 25th percentile of utilization of long-term-care facilities and services observed separately in southern and northern Ontario. It also recommended strongly that priority be given to the most undersupplied communities and regions, to bring their capacity up to that average. And it recommended that no communities or regions, even those exceeding the 75th percentile, have their capacity reduced.

There was considerable discussion on the division of Ontario into southern and northern planning groups. Many argued for equity and the application of a single planning target across the province. The commission took note of the fact that, over many years, application of the historical planning policies and practices of the Ministry of Health had resulted in greater availability and utilization (by nearly 30 percent) of long-term-care facilities and services in northern Ontario than in the province as a whole. Supporting the argument that this difference was related to need was the observation that standard mortality rates are high for all northern communities and regions. Furthermore, proportionately more elderly people (more than 30 percent) live alone in northern Ontario than in southern Ontario, possibly because there are many more private retirement homes in the more populous and prosperous south. Therefore the commission continued to recommend separate north and south planning guidelines; that applying to northern Ontario (305 beds/places per 1,000 people 75 and over) exceeded by a substantial margin the one used (215 beds/places) for southern communities and regions.

As with its study of mental health services, the commission was reluctant to get deeper into the question of how long-term-care capacity should be divided, in each community and region, among nursing homes, homes for the aged, and other facility- and community-based services. It believed that such decisions were best taken "on the ground," in this case by CCACs, which, like the proposed MHAs, comprised respected, responsible people representative of the population served and possessing the experience and knowledge necessary to make judgments about both community and regional needs and people's wishes regarding long-term care. To provide them with some rough guidance, taking current utilization as a guide and comparing the results to practices and proposals for expansion in other provinces and territories to 2003, the commission suggested that some 40 percent of each community's and region's aggregate capacity for long-term care be in long-term-care facilities; the corresponding guideline called for, on average, some 100 long-term-care beds per 1,000 people aged 75 and over.

Had it applied this guideline, Ontario would now be "in the ballpark" of the other provinces and territories. But, for reasons never disclosed, the government did not accept the commission's recommended guideline of the 50th percentile of utilization; it ended up approving the introduction of 20,000 new beds into the system. This was contrary to what the commission had favoured — namely, a phased-in approach to new long-term-care beds[16] linked to changes in the capacities of acute and complex continuing care facilities. In other words, the HSRC recommended that the immediate investment in new long-term-care beds be to replace beds displaced from the acute and complex continuing care sectors (i.e., bed reductions resulting from the elimination of ALC patients and beds currently being used for chronic care that could be provided in the long-term-care sector). It also strongly recommended that the phasing-in of the remaining increase in long-term-care places proceed in a manner consistent with the needs of the local community, by addressing the needs of those counties/regions in greatest need after dealing with the direct effects of restructuring. Ignoring its advice to take an incremental approach to the guideline that balanced the addition of "beds" and "places," the government gave priority to the addition of more institutional capacity (beds) than recommended by the HSRC. Did the institutional sector mount a more effective lobby than the home-care sector?

The HSRC also recommended that the ministry abandon its policy of basing funding on the location or provider of a service in favour of basing it on the level of care required, regardless of where and by whom it was provided. Fair implementation of this recommendation, however, is dependent on the adoption of a patient classification system common to all providers of long-term care.

Rehabilitation Care

The development of guidelines for the provision of rehabilitation services, in and out of hospital, was a particular challenge. The commission's review of the rehabilitation sector revealed an especially uneven patchwork of services that met the needs of some patient populations but failed to address the needs of others. A study completed by the Ministry of Health as the commission began its work identified some of the problems: little or no collaboration or even connection among many service providers; no policy framework on which to base funding or related decisions; inequitable access to rehabilitation services among communities/regions and population groups; lack of effective cost controls; a paucity of data on what services were being provided to whom and for what reasons, and none on the most important measure of all, the outcomes of providing rehabilitation services measured in terms of the benefits to recipients (Ontario Ministry of Health 1996). The HSRC recognized from the outset that, as with mental health, long-term and home care, the best it could do with respect to rehabilitation services, given the time and resources available, was to make a start. It could merely lay the foundation for a system of rehabilitation services and guidelines to relate the capacity of its contributors to the needs of the population. Accordingly, the focus of its review was the development of guidelines to determine the appropriate capacity of publicly funded, facility-based rehabilitation programs. It recognized that increasingly, rehabilitation services were being provided by the private sector in clinics and facilities operated on a for-profit basis. The Ministry of Health estimated in 1996 that more than $1.4 billion was being spent annually on rehabilitation services in Ontario. It spent $600 million and the Workplace Safety and Insurance Board[17] $133 million. Some of the remainder was publicly funded by other provincial ministries, including Community and Social Services, Labour, and Education and Training, but an increasing amount came from private sources in the form of expenditures made either directly by patients or indirectly by their supplementary health or automobile insurance policies. Ability to pay/affordability is an increasingly pertinent issue.

The commission began with guidelines for public-sector in-patient rehabilitation programs, starting, as it had with its studies of mental health, long-term and home care, with a discussion paper. Based on the current availability of hospital beds designated for rehabilitation patients, it proposed as a guideline the provision of 20 beds per 100,000 population to meet both regional needs (4 beds) and short- and long-term local needs (15 beds) and to accommodate patients in transition to independent living (1 bed). This guideline was predicated on increasing productivity; it foresaw hospitals providing rehabilitation services seven days a week as opposed to five and a reduction in the average length of stay, changes made possible by increasing the capacity of outpatient and in-home rehabilitation programs and transportation services to support outpatient programs.

Feedback from the field, coupled with an independent audit the HSRC had commissioned of its methodology, identified problems with these planning assumptions. The major one was that the system was too fluid to support such assumptions and, in any case, population-based guidelines for hospital rehabilitation should not be considered separately from guidelines for other providers of rehabilitation services, in particular outpatient/day hospital/outreach programs; in-home rehabilitation programs;[18] and physiotherapy, psychology, chiropractic and massage therapy offered by private rehabilitation services.[19] The provision of seven-days-a-week rehabilitation was not considered feasible either from a cost or professional-supply perspective or for clinical reasons — most patients need time away from therapy in order to heal.

Following its audit and consultations in the field, the commission revised its guideline to provide 25 rehabilitation hospital beds or places per 100,000 people, allocated according to regional (4 beds) and local (21 beds) needs, the latter to be divided between patients requiring short-term (14 days or less) and long-term care. Consistent with its conviction that decisions are best made by those on the ground with expertise and experience, the HSRC recommended that the Ministry of Health facilitate the development of local networks of providers of rehabilitation services and that such networks include both for-profit providers and CCACs. It also recommended the creation of a province-wide network, funded by the government, to address the policy-oriented challenge of pulling together a genuine system of rehabilitation services.

The ministry endorsed the commission's proposed planning guideline. It agreed that its implementation should be a gradual, planned, "systematic rebalancing" of facility- and community-based rehabilitation services.[20] It rejected, however, the HSRC's classification of "local" and "regional" beds and confirmed its intention to continue using its historical terminology and data reporting definitions[21] and processes.[22]

Subacute Care

Subacute care was a particularly contentious topic. Used in a number of American and other jurisdictions, this category of care is designed for ALC patients — those who no longer need acute care but are not yet ready for discharge without some continuing care; it excludes those patients who do require complex continuing care, rehabilitation or long-term care. The HSRC concluded that subacute beds should be created in Ontario, for several reasons. The continued use of empty physical facilities in hospitals containing a substantial number of closed acute-care and other beds made sense from the perspective of making the best use of capital and operating funds and making the most efficient use of available qualified workers and existing hospital infrastructure. Another compelling reason was that the availability of such beds and appropriate services would reduce the danger of patients being discharged too early and ease their transition to other forms and sites of care or to their homes and communities.

The commission appointed a task force of consumers, hospital and long-term-care representatives and health professionals (including physicians) to review the situation in other jurisdictions, define subacute care and produce a discussion paper to provide a focus for consultations with those potentially affected throughout Ontario. That paper described subacute care as three to five hours of medical/nursing services per day, plus rehabilitation, laboratory and related services, on either a short-term (less than 14 days) or long-term basis. It suggested that a minimum of 14 such beds be available per 100,000 people.

The report of this task force received much attention and generated a good deal of heated argument, not so much within the commission as among those potentially affected by the creation of the new category of beds. The hospitals did not want to see subacute care established as a distinct category, fearing that their responsibility for the care of large numbers of ALC patients would continue but would be funded at a lower rate. They also feared the creation of private, American-style free-standing subacute-care facilities, which would compete with them (and with other facilities such as nursing homes offering subacute care) for government funding. The community-based providers of home care and nursing-home care were concerned that subacute hospital beds would diminish the "business" coming their way. Opinions were expressed about how subacute care should be defined. Many respondents emphasized the importance of making clear where rehabilitation services did and did not apply. In all of this the ministry stayed quiet, but it was clear to the commission that the bureaucrats were less than keen on the idea of creating this or any other new category of hospital bed.

On the basis of the feedback it received, the HSRC considered the possibility of placing subacute beds in different locations based on its review of a number of factors, including the quality of care available, keeping disruption of care to a minimum, patient characteristics, community needs, physical-plant capacities and critical mass. Subacute care could be located within:

> *full-service acute-care hospitals,* by converting inpatient beds to subacute beds and aggregating them within a subacute-care program
> *complex continuing care and/or rehabilitation hospitals,* by converting inpatient beds to subacute beds within a subacute-care program

> *long-term-care facilities,* by converting long-term-care beds to subacute-care beds
> *free standing subacute-care facilities,* by converting acute or complex continuing care hospitals or long-term-care facilities into subacute-care facilities or by building new subacute-care facilities

In the end, the commission concluded that introducing subacute care in Ontario was a good idea but that such care should be exclusively hospital-based. Confining it to hospitals would minimize patient transfers to other sites and avoid unnecessary discontinuities in care. Also, maintaining this category of patient in the same facility would result in more productive use of the hospital's infrastructure. Accordingly, the HSRC recommended that the ministry endorse its definition of subacute care and the guideline that 13 beds per 100,000 population be established in hospitals for this purpose. It also recommended that the funding of subacute care be in the order of $200 per day and be provided to hospitals in an envelope separate from their global budget. After a long silence, the commission was informed that the ministry had not accepted its recommendation.

ACTION ON RECOMMENDATIONS

The greatest frustration for the commission was the government's reaction (or lack thereof) to its many recommendations relating to planning guidelines and implementation strategies for mental health, long-term, subacute and home care and rehabilitation. This was as true for the recommendations presented in the consolidated report of April 1998 (*Change and Transition*) as it was for the several restructuring reports concerning specific communities and regions, beginning with Thunder Bay as early as October 4, 1996.

Nobody can claim that these recommendations were sprung on the government or on any other party; their evolution, with the commission conducting in-depth and very public studies of each issue, was designed to avoid surprises. Formal progress reports were provided to the minister on a quarterly basis. Ministerial officials were closely involved and consulted by the commission's staff as each study progressed. Yet invariably, as the HSRC's restructuring *Notices* and *Directions* and summary reports were published, and its recommendations specifically drawn to the attention of the ministry, the initial reaction was dead silence. It was disconcerting to the commissioners that the principal beneficiary and inheritor of the commission's mantle, after a long, intense, time-consuming process culminating in the release of a report of vital concern to the community, reacted as if their recommendations had been dropped into a deep, dark hole. Frequently the ministry's response would come to the commission only after it had been requested formally, sometimes repeatedly, in letters from the chair to the minister. Everybody came to appreciate the deep frustration of "working with the government."

It is difficult to determine what proportion of the commission's recommendations were accepted and acted upon. Things are still happening nine years after the commission first convened. Certainly once the government became confident, in the spring of 1998, that it could afford to reinvest substantial sums in long-term and home care (and that politically it could ill afford *not* to do so), decisions were taken to increase dramatically the capacity of these two community-based services. But other cost-neutral and even cost-saving recommendations, like providing funding envelopes to Mental Health Implementation Task Forces and creating the category of hospital-based subacute beds, were eventually rejected. Others were said to be "under consideration," meaning that they had been put in limbo. Worse than that, many recommendations were simply ignored. The commission was never directly and only rarely indirectly given reasons why so many of its recommendations, those related to both hospital restructuring and reinvestment in community-based services and subsequently system building, did not find favour with the ministry or with the government in general.

Looking at the "big picture" in 2005, one sees that there has been more progress than was apparent at the commission's sunset. Some 20,000 new long-term-care beds are online and the capacity of home care and other non-institutional providers has increased, though by how much it is hard to say. Although the jury is still out on whether the government will act on their advice, the Mental Health Implementation Task Forces brought together providers and others to develop coherent plans, involving many institutions and agencies, to provide more comprehensive health and social services to people and families burdened with mental health problems. Good things are happening in rehabilitation; networks of providers have been established, the contributions of rehabilitation to the care continuum are being studied, changes are being made in education and training programs, and research in the whole field has been stimulated. Home care is alive, well, much expanded and prominent on every provincial and even the national radar screen. The idea of subacute care is being discussed openly, despite the fact that it is still stuck in some official dead-letter office in Queen's Park. On all counts there are grounds for cautious optimism.

On the downside, the commission's carefully calculated targets for Ontario's bed capacity in 2003 have not been met. There are long waiting lists for acute care, mainly because the government continues to fund hospital capacity inadequately. There continues to be uncertainty about funding for home care appropriate to the demands placed on it throughout the range of services offered. Capital investments out of the public purse, whether in buildings or high-technology equipment, remain severely constrained, and hospitals and communities are increasingly using scarce resources to compete with one another in fundraising campaigns for the matching dollars required.

From the commission's perspective, much less was accomplished than could have been, during and immediately following the period 1996-2000, to restructure hospitals, jump-start integration of the silos and foster the creation of a genuine health care system in Ontario. A tremendous amount of work and energy was devoted to the commission. It addressed an unparalleled range of difficult topics, many of which had never been seriously considered before. A good deal of political capital was put at risk in its very creation and more was put at risk throughout its duration, capital that has earned much less return than it ought to have done. The people of Ontario are paying the price for that, in terms of ongoing discontinuities in care for patients and higher costs than necessary for taxpayers (i.e., lower productivity). This can be measured against the fact that Ontario's health care consumers and taxpayers still do not have access to information on how well or how poorly health care is being provided in their province. Neither their government nor anybody else can answer fundamental questions that everybody wants answered: Are we getting our money's worth? Are we making progress toward a real system of health care? Are we standing still or sliding backwards?

NOTES

1. The Resource Planning Group, was the primary group to advise on facilities-planning issues.
2. For 1993 to 1996.
3. Some progress has been made in recent years, particularly in the rehabilitation and complex continuing care sectors. CIHI has developed a National Rehabilitation Reporting System (NRS) and a data set for adult in-patient rehabilitation services in Canada. The project is focused on collecting, processing and analyzing data on adult in-patient rehabilitation services; supporting management decision-making at the facility, regional and provincial/territorial levels; facilitating provincial/territorial and national comparative reporting; and supporting related research. Effective October 1, 2003, the Ministry of Health mandated the implementation of the NRS for the reporting of adult in-patient rehabilitation activity, with every patient being assessed at admission, discharge and follow-up (optional) using the NRS tool. Some progress is also being made within the complex continuing care sector. For example, the Minimum Data Set (MDS) – which serves as the mandated assessment tool within the sector – is providing a basis for development of a centralized database in that sector. In addition, the OHA Report Card Project now includes a core set of performance indicators for the rehabilitation and complex continuing care sectors.
4. The other report, released in 1987 by the Liberal government, *Building Community Support for People: A Plan for Mental Health in Ontario* (the Graham report), established key principles for mental health reform. The 1994 report, *Putting People First*, was developed under the NDP government and announced a 10-year mental health reform strategy.
5. The HSRC recommended nine MHITFs, in North East (North Bay), North West (Lakehead), Central West (Hamilton), Simcoe (Penetanguishene), South West (London/St. Thomas), Central East (Kingston), East (Brockville), Durham (Whitby), and Toronto (Queen Street).
6. The Ministry of Health established MHITFs in Northeastern Ontario, Northwestern Ontario, Champlain Region, Southeast Region, Central South Region (Hamilton), Toronto-Peel, Central East (Whitby), Central East (Penetanguishene) and Southwest.
7. The substitution of home care for in-hospital care is essential to hospital restructuring. The HSRC's official definition of postacute home care was health services provided in the patient's home within 30 days of an in-patient or same-day surgical discharge.
8. Available at http://www.hc-sc.gc.ca/english/hca2003/accord.html (accessed July 5, 2005). The "basket of services" for short-term acute home care included mental health and end-of-life care. The first ministers agreed that they would provide "first-dollar coverage" for these services, access to which would be based on assessed need, and that by 2006 available services *could* include nursing/professional services, pharmaceuticals and medical equipment/supplies, support for personal care needs and case management.
9. Determined by adding up six modalities of long-term care.
10. Each of the utilization measures for each modality of care was translated into a measurement of equivalent long-term-care places per 1,000 population (75+). Although more sensitive population age groups (e.g., 0-19, 19-44, 45-64, 65-74, 75-84, 85+) would have been preferable, their use was not supported by the data available.
11. MDS/RUGS III is the patient classification system used by nursing staff and other health providers to conduct assessments of individuals in designated beds, whether in freestanding chronic or long-term-care facilities or in hospitals. The data are collected using the Resident Assessment

Instrument (RAI) Minimum Data Set (MDS 2.0), © interRAI 1997, 1999, modified by CIHI for use in the Continuing Care Reporting System. The RAI MDS 2.0© clinical assessment tool consists of more than 500 data elements, including demographics, cognitive and behavioural data, physical functioning, medication use, nutritional status, and special treatments and procedures. In April 2003 the Ontario Ministry of Health mandated data submission on chronic care patients in Ontario for inclusion in the Ontario Chronic Care Patient System.

12 Ironically, it was not used by the Alberta government for funding purposes.
13 Physical Function Reduced; Behavioural Problems; Impaired Cognition; Clinically Complex; Special Care; Extensive Services; Special Rehabilitation.
14 Clinically Complex; Special Care; Extensive Services.
15 The HSRC gave first priority to the availability of palliative services in an individual's place of residence (e.g., home, long-term-care facility, complex continuing care facility). The inclusion of palliative-care beds in the complex continuing care guideline recognized the need to provide some institutional palliative-care programs within a hospital setting.
16 Initially using the HSRC bed guidelines for planning.
17 Formerly the Workers' Compensation Board.
18 Provided by, for example, the Arthritis Society Consultation and Therapy Service (Ontario) and the Community Occupational Therapists Association.
19 Some of these services are billable to provincial health plans; others are covered out-of-pocket or through extended health insurance plans and/or provincial workers' insurance programs.
20 The HSRC suggested that the new planning guideline would impact differently on communities depending on their current bed ratios. Communities with higher bed ratios would lose beds toward the benchmark, as bed numbers of communities with lower bed ratios would increase toward the benchmark.
21 The HSRC had proposed the term "local" to designate beds for patients from the immediate community, whether for short-term or long-term care, and "regional" to designate beds for patients with more complex needs drawn to regional centres for specialized care. The ministry's terms "general" and "specialized" remained.
22 The Ministry of Health confirmed this decision in a letter to hospitals in the summer of 2002.

CHAPTER 6

THE RESTRUCTURING OF A HEALTH-SERVICES SYSTEM

Although very much on the minds of the commissioners from day one, the heavy demands of hospital restructuring limited the investment of time and resources that could be made, during the first half of the HSRC's mandate, in the development of strategies to foster the creation of a genuine health care system in Ontario. By late 1998, however, the corner had been turned on phase I. The approaches and methodologies applicable to hospital restructuring were by then well developed and tested. The commission's two analytical teams, headed by Peter Finkle and Mario Tino, although still pressed by the volume of work to be done within tight, self-imposed timelines, were confident they could meet the timetable for hospital restructuring. Much work remained to be done only in two northern communities, North Bay and Sault Ste. Marie, and in the large regional municipality of Niagara. In addition, the complex review of small rural, northern and remote hospitals then well underway was yet to be completed preparatory to the commission's issuing its decisions[1] on how best to organize them into networks in accordance with the broad policy framework established by the Ministry of Health. *Notices* and final *Directions* had been issued for the hospitals in the "big eight" communities,[2] those allocated the largest proportion of funds from the ministry's hospital envelope, although additional work leading to supplementary *Directions* was still to be done in Ottawa and Toronto.

Some of the commissioners felt ill prepared for the new system orientation and broad policy decision-making required in phase II. While phase I had consisted largely of fulfilling the mandate of making decisions about hospital restructuring on a community-by-community basis, the expectations of the government and the "field" with respect to phase II were less clear.

Although the commissioners and staff members appreciated the urgency of beginning phase II, there were still tough decisions to be made before hospital restructuring could be completed; there was de facto competition between the two phases for resources and time at the commission table. Some thought the HSRC should spend the majority of its remaining time on tracking implementation of the *Directions* issued during phase I. Others were keen to get on with the system-building work that had attracted them to the commission in the first place.

All of this was coincident with a number of changes — a new deputy minister, the government's reducing the HSRC's role to a purely advisory one and the departure of Mark Rochon. Finding and recruiting a new chief executive officer claimed first priority. The task was to find someone quickly with the ability, credibility and flexibility to handle ongoing work plus the interest and capability to shift the commission's focus, leading it into the different kind of work necessary in phase II. Peggy Leatt, who had just completed a second term as chair of the Department of Health Administration at the University of Toronto, brought to this challenge a strong reputation in the academic, research and policy arenas and extensive knowledge derived from research on integrated heath systems (IHSs) — a key element in the HSRC's vision of Ontario's future health care system.

The shifting of gears necessary to address the mandate of phase II required a change in the culture and perspectives of the HSRC. A number of factors were involved. The commissioners were getting tired, but there was much yet to do and little time in which to do it. They had bonded — faced the "enemy" together and for the most part succeeded. They had enjoyed using their power to make things happen. They had been confronted by challenges to the courts and had had their decision-making processes, *Directions* and authority affirmed.[3] Some commissioners and staff members had settled into the routines of hospital restructuring, the development and implementation of which had taken so much of their time. Now they had to shift from a familiar analytical role to the broader and far less defined one necessitated by the policy issues entailed in system-building. Some commissioners were eager for the new challenge, others not. Some staff members, with the end of the HSRC clearly in sight, began looking for new jobs. Others clearly relished their new roles.

But given that time was indeed running out, the commissioners soon reached consensus that it was now or never — time to tackle phase II. The first challenge was to decide where to start. Where could the HSRC make the greatest impact? Of all the policy issues it could work on, which were the most important? Which had the most potential to move the yardsticks the farthest toward the development of a genuine system of health services?

In order to prioritize any future projects, the commissioners sought to gain a better sense of public attitudes — the perceptions, degree of support, and priorities of people on the street with regard to change, renewal and repair of their health care system. The commission posed a number of questions:

> How does the public perceive the current health care system, and how should public perceptions be factored into the planning of reforms?
> What are the best approaches to changing perceptions and creating fresh insights in order to enhance the potential for constructive change?
> What do the public consider the real priorities in health care reform?
> What are the best ways to engage the public and providers in open dialogue that will develop and broaden a consensus for change?
> What are the political and other obstacles to better coordination and integration of health services, and how can they be overcome?
> What political and other issues affecting nongovernmental stakeholders must be taken into account when planning and implementing health care reforms?

The HSRC "kick-started" phase II by exploring these questions in four steps:

(1) A retreat to plan for phase II and reach agreement on a general approach to addressing work in this area.
(2) Assessment of the public (consumer) environment, analysis of public opinion on current health-system reforms, and review of public behaviour, perceptions and priorities.
(3) Meetings with policy and research experts (a policy forum organized by the Queen's University School of Policy Studies) to determine the positioning of future changes in the health care system and with four previous deputy ministers[4] to get their advice on what HSRC should/could do in its last few months.
(4) Assessment of the provider environment based on roundtable discussions with key stakeholder groups to solicit feedback on what the priorities and next steps should be in reforming Ontario's health care system.

COMMISSION RETREAT

A retreat for commissioners and staff, led by Leatt, who had taken over as chief executive officer in September, was held in late 1998. The goal was to develop the commission's approach to the challenge of converting the notorious "field of silos" into a system in which the contributions of all the many providers of health services would be smoothly coordinated. The conclusions and recommendations emanating from the retreat were debated at a formal commission meeting in December when a plan of action was approved. At the same meeting a task force was created to begin building a strategy for the development of what the commission agreed should be one of its top priorities: a health information management system — something that was central to moving beyond silos to a true system.[5] The HSRC staff set out to identify the elements involved in developing strategy for another key step, reform of primary care, the gateway through which most people access the spectrum of health services available in Ontario.

VISION OF THE SYSTEM

Despite its preoccupation with hospital restructuring during phase I, the commission had also laid the groundwork for system building, by developing, discussing and widely disseminating its vision of a health-services system. A preliminary statement of that vision was disseminated in January 1997, as the working hypothesis the HSRC followed as it proceeded with restructuring (HSRC 1997a). It was also used as a foundation for further development, in phase II, of a policy framework and strategic steps to foster the creation of such a system. The vision had two principal characteristics. The first, as illustrated in figure 3, was a shift in the focus of health services from one akin to the Ptolemaic view of the solar system, with hospitals at the centre, to the Copernican model that replaced it, in which the providers in the system revolve around patients and the populations from which they come.

The second characteristic, as illustrated in figure 4, was reorganization of the providers of health services into integrated systems. The commission had in mind the desirability of the ministry's devolution to IHSs the bulk of operational responsibility for meeting the needs of their communities, in accordance with the

Figure 3
CURRENT AND FUTURE MODELS OF HEALTH REFORM

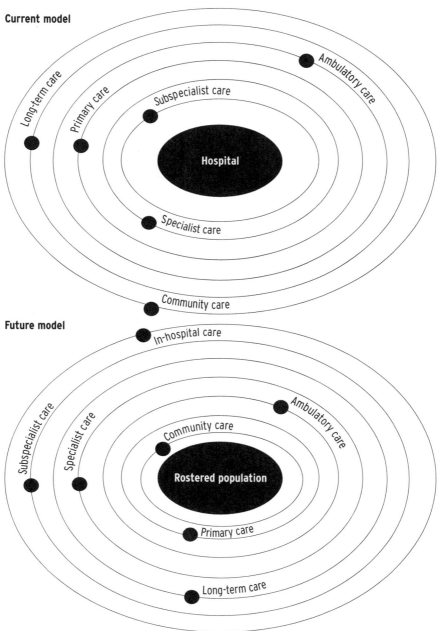

Source: Adapted, with permission, from a presentation by Roger S. Hunt, president and chief executive officer, Greater Rochester Health System, to the Annual Fellows Dinner of the Canadian College of Health Service Executives, November 4, 1996 (HSRC 1997a, 3).

Figure 4
INTEGRATED HEALTH SYSTEMS

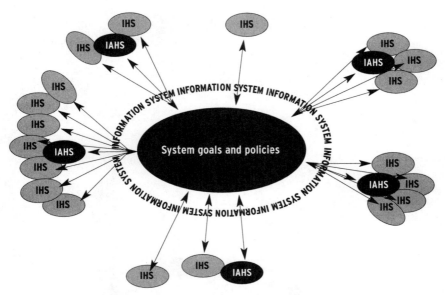

IHS = Integrated health system   IAHS = Integrated academic health system

Source: HSRC (1997a, 4).

vision, goals and policies clearly defined by the government — that is, its governance of the system as a whole. Funding from the public purse would flow to the IHSs on a risk-adjusted capitation basis. Accountability would be supported by a comprehensive health information system linking the system's central governance to the users and providers of the services. A dozen characteristics of the IHSs in the commission's vision are described in table 3. The commission's vision statement was widely distributed and feedback on the concept and statement invited from both health care providers and members of the public.

Despite its repeated efforts to "talk up" the significance of the vision statement and the provocative concepts embedded in it, the HSRC was unable to engage the full attention of the government, the spectrum of health care providers, the media or the public. While most of the feedback it received was thoughtful and useful, none was the product of the intense debate and widespread discussion the commission had hoped to stimulate by distributing a

Table 3

ESSENTIAL CHARACTERISTICS OF A GENUINELY INTEGRATED HEALTH SYSTEM

Common vision: All sectors and every constituent institution and organization share a common vision.	**Shared goals, priorities and performance standards**: Sectors have shared goals, priorities and performance standards to optimize accessibility and quality of service.	**Backdrop of provincial legislation policy and standards:** Policies and plans are set by the Ministry of Health and are adjusted periodically in response to evaluation of the system's performance in achieving the ministry's goals and objectives.
Focus on population health: The system's focus is population health as well as individual health.	**Balance between health care and population health:** The emphasis and resource allocation between the long-term goal of enhancing the population's health and the immediate imperatives of diagnosing and treating illness are balanced over time.	**Common information system:** A shared information system provides comprehensive, up-to-date and accurate data in order to plan, coordinate and operate the IHS.
Vertical and horizontal integration: The diverse institutions and organizations that offer the same type of services are organized horizontally into sectors. These sectors are vertically integrated so they operate together within each region.	**Diversity in developing strategic alliances that support greater integration and efficiencies:** The system fosters local, district, and regional initiative and diversity, and achieves horizontal and vertical coordination among institutions, organizations and sectors.	**Shared accountability:** Fiscal envelopes and purchaser-provider concepts (among others) are used to achieve specific objectives and safeguard particular services such as mental health and children's services.
Incentives: Incentives are created and disincentives removed to encourage providers and consumers to strive for good health.	**Leadership:** Professionals and others provide strong leadership and commitment to meet current and evolving health care needs.	**Capitation funding:** Envelope funding allows organizations to meet the total health needs of a defined or rostered population, and to operate within the financial limits of individuals, the public purse and the provincial economy.

statement that, it believed, had the potential to lay the foundation for a health-services system recast to meet the needs and aspirations of Ontarians into the twenty-first century. It was as if the development and declaration of a vision of a health-services system was an academic[6] exercise without real consequence to the financial and control issues in health care that preoccupy most people.

Nevertheless, throughout the early part of 1997 the commission did receive a good deal of commentary on its working hypothesis and, as a result, shortened the vision statement, gave it a sharper focus and made it more "user-friendly." The HSRC was heartened to find that the fundamental concepts embedded in its vision seemed to be accepted or at least not seriously challenged. Those concepts consisted of shifting health care's orientation from providers to patients and populations, and linking, through a comprehensive health information system, the governance responsibilities of government with those of service delivery by community-based, vertically integrated health care systems. The commission concluded that its vision was appropriate with respect to both restructuring hospitals and the broader challenge of fostering the development of a health-services system.

While the HSRC continued to keep its vision clearly in focus, it recognized that government-sanctioned development of IHSs in Ontario, however desirable, was just not going to happen soon. There were too many constraints in the political environment and everybody had as much as they could manage on their plates with the changes then underway. So as a precursor to developing its work plan for phase II, the HSRC concluded that although it would not advocate for the formal establishment of IHSs in the near term, it should retain this as a long-term goal. The challenge, then, was to determine which opportunities held the greatest potential for building on current reforms, continuing to rebalance the various components/elements with the system and enhancing continuity of care.

Neither was the commission under any illusion that intensifying its foray into health policy in phase II would be easy or that the results would be eagerly received and quickly implemented. It did perceive, however, an opportunity to contribute innovative, well-documented and well-argued proposals for change that would, at the very least, lay out before the various players a set of priorities, together with strategies they could use to test their chances of making change successfully. For the government the tests would be primarily those of assessing the cost — in political as well as financial terms — of taking on the entrenched interests likely to be fiercely resistant to change. For the other players, mainly representatives of those entrenched interests, the tests would be of how the proposed strategies would affect their power, influence, incomes and, particularly with respect to hospitals, relative autonomy from the constraints of systemization — of having to work collaboratively with other providers of health care.

Although (given a long-term perspective) the need persisted, by late 1998 the volume and shrillness of cries for change had been diminished by virtue of the fact that Ontario's economy had picked up. The government's coffers were filling at a rate that forecast the promised end to deficit financing and permitted relaxation of the intense, unrelenting drive to reduce spending. The third of the reductions of 7 percent in hospital funding scheduled for 1998-99 was not applied. While the improved economic circumstances diminished the commission's opportunity to stimulate change through policy development, they did not eliminate it. There were many people, in and out of government, who had lots of experience with economic ups and downs and who knew that the sharp spur of lean times would return, and sooner than later. Many saw that, without change, especially in the rate of growth of its appetite for money, health care's problems would only intensify as time went on.

Among the most influential potential change agents was Elizabeth Witmer, the minister of health. Although as one of the government's most senior members she was bound to and driven by its political agenda, Witmer appreciated the need for fundamental change in the organization and delivery of health services and knew that a policy vacuum had long existed within her ministry. Her authority[7] and her willingness to advocate for new ways of doing things constituted the commission's best opportunity to make a difference as it set about tackling phase II of its mandate.

Another opportunity was presented by the growing and increasingly vocal dissatisfaction of providers of home care, long-term care and other community-based services, who saw in the commission a potential champion in their long campaign to achieve major-league status and funding. During phase I the HSRC had made it clear that sensible restructuring of acute-care hospitals was dependent on the government's reinvesting the money saved (and more) in community-based care. The wisdom of this advice was not lost on the media and the general public, who rewarded the providers of these services with heightened visibility, which increased the probability, in the commission's opinion, that its policy advice on system building would fall on more receptive ears.

But the barriers remained more or less constant: the bureaucracy and the vested interests, particularly hospitals and health care professionals. The common feature was nothing more than simple resistance to change. Dean Aberman's quip about changing light bulbs[8] applies — to doctors, yes, but also to many other professional groups and institutions (and to governments).

PUBLIC OPINION

Before deciding on the priority of projects, the HSRC wished to gain a better sense of the public's attitudes — the perceptions, degree of support and priorities of people on the street regarding their health care system. It commissioned a study leading to a report titled *Public Behaviour, Perceptions and Priorities in the Health Sector: An Overview* (HayGroup 1999), which summarized the results of an analysis of Canada Health Monitor (CHM) surveys taken over a 10-year period. These public-opinion surveys revealed that from the mid-1980s to the mid-1990s a growing proportion of Ontarians were dissatisfied with the health care system and concerned about its future. They showed that Ontarians believed that their access to health services had become more restricted and that there was a rapidly growing need for home care. The surveys also showed that Ontarians were ready for reform. In particular, there appeared to be an understanding among the public that advances in medical technology and knowledge, changes in people's expectations and preferences, and changing demographic trends called for modernization of the ways in which health services were delivered. In addition, the surveys indicated that the views of respected leaders in the health care field, especially physicians and nurses, had a strong influence on public opinion.

EXPERT ADVICE ON THE PROCESS OF CHANGE

A policy forum of academic and research experts in the health sector was organized on behalf of the HSRC by the Queen's University School of Policy Studies (see appendix 4 for a list of participants), leading to the report *Path Dependency, Positioning and Legitimacy* (Queen's University School of Policy Studies 1999).[9] This discussion brought together representatives of the HSRC and a small group of international experts on the interface between politics and health care. It confirmed much of what had been identified in the review of CHM surveys — that Ontario residents were ready for reforms that would ensure their access to high-quality, dependable health services and incorporate community-based care into a properly coordinated health-services system. There was consensus that any future process leading to change would have to reassure Ontarians that health care reforms would be both "made in

Ontario" and aimed at improving public access to high-quality health services rather than cutting costs.

As for the question of how best to design the reform agenda, the expert panel was very clear:

> The change process should avoid steps that could be perceived by the public as reducing each person's sense of control over his or her health. Proposed changes should incorporate reforms that enhance informed consumer choice, such as: development of a consumers' information service to prepare consumer-friendly data on the health services available to Ontarians; creation of a health-services ombudsman with wide jurisdiction to address legitimate consumer complaints about systemic problems outside the purview of any one group of providers or institutions; and proposals related to service availability, hours of access, information sources, patient and client convenience, and so on to increase public confidence and provide "customer service" incentives to providers.

> Proposed changes should be made clear, explicit and specific, and they should not be presented in the abstract or in the language of theory. For example, while terms such as "integrated system" and "continuum of care" describe important concepts understood by health planners and policy-makers, the public is more interested in the specific results of the application of such concepts and how they might affect the provision of health services to men, women and children on the street. Therefore, any consultation should focus on clear, specific statements of goals and objectives and on strategies to achieve them instead of abstract principles or aspirations. Specific proposals for broad public debate should take the form of reports to the government from the HSRC (or other advisory bodies) and should not originate with government itself.

> Reform proposals should include descriptions of clearly defined benefits or gains to offset the pain that people inevitably associate with change.

> Every proposed change should reinforce the spirit and intent of the *Canada Health Act* and its five principles applicable to publicly funded health care: universality, accessibility, comprehensiveness, portability and public administration of the insurance plan itself.

> A "big bang" approach to health care reform should be avoided. The creation of an integrated health care system should be an evolutionary process in which changes are incremental and approached through

several alternative, parallel pathways signposted with clear incentives for both citizens and providers to shift from the old path to a new one.[10]
> Support by health-service providers for initiatives in system integration is critical. Physicians remain the most respected voice in forming public opinion about health care, followed by hospitals, nurses and providers of community care. When faced with proposals, members of the public will seek providers' views on integration and will be more influenced by them than by government, planning bodies (like the HSRC) or anybody else.
> The adoption of any new model should be preceded by a consultative process that seeks to establish as wide a consensus as possible around the change(s) proposed. Any change forced on an unconvinced public and resistant providers through a unilateral, binding, government-mandated process will not succeed.
> The consultation process should be conducted by an advisory body separate from government. For example, a community-based citizens' panel[11] could be struck and charged with seeking reaction to a proposed change. Such a panel would comprise a diversity of lay and expert citizens asked to bring their best judgment to the issues and to not represent any particular stakeholder. Ideally, the result would be a group of apolitical spokespeople for the benefits resulting from proposed changes leading to a more seamless, integrated system.
> Each proposed change should be accompanied by a multifaceted strategic and tactical communications plan, to launch debate effectively and avoid its derailment by comments from the media and vested interests.
> Building momentum for change from the ground up is vitally important in the formation of broad consensus from the consultative process.

ROUND-TABLE DISCUSSIONS

Phase II began with a series of round-table discussions by leading health-service providers in Ontario. The objective was to gain a sense of what well-informed insiders believed should be the next steps in health reform. A total of 18 such discussions were convened. Among the priority issues consistently identified were:[12]

> articulating and communicating a *vision of health reform* for Ontario
> creating an accessible *health information management* infrastructure
> making *primary health care* the foundation of future reforms by positioning it as the "connector" to all other elements in the system
> *enhancing integration* by eliminating the silo effect perpetuated by the traditional boundaries between caregivers
> *aligning incentives* for both providers and consumers of health care to stimulate "systems" thinking and behaviour and improve accountability at all levels

But the consensus that emerged around these issues as common themes did not necessarily equate with a common understanding or interpretation of their meaning. Their relative priority varied by provider and discussion group. Neither was there agreement on the optimum strategy to support them. Nevertheless, these themes were adopted by the commission as the basis for the consultations and analyses it undertook subsequently.

Three studies — on public opinion, on how best to approach the public with proposals for change and on the opinions of providers — formed the necessary background and context for the commission to identify the priorities, scope and pace of phase II. The results made it abundantly clear that the public and health professions saw the need for change. They shared the belief that health care would be improved by restructuring beyond hospitals. The HSRC accepted the message that, provided the foreseen benefits were easily understood and seen to outweigh the risks, the public would be supportive of changes leading to greater continuity of care and integration of health-service providers.

The commission then set to work on the task of (1) formulating health care policies capable of winning acceptance by the diverse interest groups affected, and (2) developing implementation strategies capable of convincing the government of the political and financial practicality of those policies.

HEALTH INFORMATION MANAGEMENT

The HSRC turned its immediate attention to the need for a comprehensive health information management system. This was central to all potential reforms of the health care system, both as a whole and in all of its many elements. Unless complete and reliable data are available on the relationship between the costs of "doing business" in different environments (hospital care, primary care, specialist care, home care, rehabilitation care, etc.) and the comparative benefits to recipients, then it will never be possible to determine whether any given change is improving things, making them worse or having no effect at all.

This was every commissioner's highest priority. Decisions at all levels (from policy development, through care and treatment, to informed patient choice) would be far better informed if comprehensive data were available and used throughout the health care system. People are shocked to learn how little evidence-based decision-making takes place in health care. The commission was convinced that health information and its effective management constituted the *fundamental enabler* of all changes affecting health care. Without information, there is neither the knowledge nor the accountability to support the effective governance or efficient operation of any enterprise, including health care.

In the late 1990s Ontario lacked the fundamental information necessary to integrate the work of its many individual and institutional care providers, and the capacity to exchange and share that information. Health-service providers cannot deliver coordinated care to their patients without proper communication across the care continuum with regard to their diagnoses, treatments, progress and specific care requirements. The problem is partly technical. Many providers, especially those in the community-care and long-term-care sectors, have been slow to acquire and incorporate computers and information communication tools into their daily operations, thus hampering the collection and sharing of information. During the commission's mandate, most such providers attributed this shortcoming to the inadequacy of government funding, a justification the HSRC did not fully buy. Determined leadership is every bit as important as money. Up-to-date information technology is vital to efficient management and customer satisfaction in any modern enterprise. The hard fact is that neither government nor the caregiving organizations themselves have given this enough priority.

Although by 1998 a number of organizations and institutional and individual providers throughout the spectrum of health services had begun to invest in the technology and personnel to support their operations, there was no overarching, guiding framework to coordinate their investments or facilitate the sharing of information. The commission quickly discovered that the chief reason why so little of the existing health information could be shared was that there were few common standards for data, communication protocols or even identifiers (for care recipients or providers). The Canadian Institute for Health Information (CIHI) had established a number of standards for in-patient services and was working on data and communication standards for outpatient and some out-of-hospital services. But elsewhere in the system such data and communication standards as existed were those of the myriad commercial vendors of hardware and software. Each vendor, of course, stood to profit from its product's becoming the standard and, for proprietary reasons, was not much interested in compatibility.

Another problem was the absence of a comprehensive legislative framework in Ontario to safeguard the privacy of individual health records, or even to establish ownership of and control over access to each record. The longer this policy vacuum continued, the commission perceived, the harder it would become to remedy, as the "local solutions" of computer-literate health-service providers became more and more deeply embedded.

All of these issues were addressed by a task force[13] established by the HSRC in late 1998 under the leadership of Michael Guerriere, executive vice-president of the University Health Network. The task force comprised experts in information management from Ontario and elsewhere in Canada with experience in the challenges faced by hospitals and other major players in health care, as well as representatives of the provincial government (the Ministry of Health and the Management Board). Its mandate was to define a framework for the immediate establishment of capacity for the management of health information. The group focused not so much on supporting computer and communication technologies as on defining and getting a handle on the management of health information — that is, the data and, after analysis, knowledge needed by providers, consumers, managers and the government to enhance decision-making by rooting it more firmly in objectively produced evidence.

A little over six months later, in June 1999, the HSRC submitted to the minister the *Ontario Health Information Management Action Plan* (HSRC 1999b). This set out a comprehensive strategy for building the capacity to collect and manage the information necessary to preserve the health of the population, give consumers access to the information they need in order to make health care choices and provide the spectrum of health services efficiently and effectively. Central to the commission's 22 recommendations was a call for strong, informed leadership — for consistent, coherent *governance* of the long process of building a system of health information management, a process that would be much longer than the time horizon of most governments. The commission recommended that an arm's-length body, much like the HSRC itself, be established and funded to provide that governance; it estimated that it would cost between $500 and $700 million over three years to improve:

> > customer information — the creation of a consumer-information hotline and Web site to dispense advice and answer questions relating to health and health services
> > the delivery of health services at the point of care — initiatives to support, with evidence, the decisions and practices of health care providers, including province-wide drug and laboratory information
> > the management of health services — improved forecasting of needs (including the need for health professionals) and analysis of the outcome of the myriad interactions between consumers and health-service providers

Aware that this was an ambitious and expensive agenda, especially from the perspective of bureaucrats fearful of losing control, the HSRC advised the minister that developing the capacity to collect, analyze and distribute health information to providers and consumers alike was the priority for improving the health care system. It had to be done. Furthermore, implementation of the action plan offered the greatest potential return on the investment to consumers, providers, managers and the government. The HSRC also pointed out the costs of inaction. Ontario was clearly behind many provinces in coming to grips with health information management. Some $500 million was being spent annually in Ontario, throughout the system, on information and computing technologies, the great majority of it wasted in the absence of strong, coordinated leadership. The commission emphasized its conviction that without effective health information management no real reform of health services was possible. In the absence of convincing evidence, drawn from credible data, to counter the doleful predictions of physicians and other vested interests, as well as media stories about patients dying on gurneys while waiting for care, the status quo would prevail.

Despite the power of these arguments and the vigour of their presentation, during the last few months of the commission's mandate it became clear that the action plan and its recommendations were not going to be accepted. A couple of meetings with the minister and the deputy minister[14] made it clear that while they and others praised the report, the government was simply not in a position to free up the millions of dollars needed to create such a system. What they failed to say was that the government and its bureaucracy were not prepared to let an "outside" body take control. The commissioners believed this to be a much greater obstacle than the money.

Subsequently, at a meeting convened by the chair and the chief executive officer of the commission, four former deputy ministers of health[15] confirmed that health information management was a vital issue and that the commission's recommendations were indeed sound; at the same time, all four said the recommendations stood no chance of being implemented, because "an investment in an initiative of this type is neither exciting nor flashy enough to catch the attention of the most important people — voters."

Changes to the design and management of health information systems continue to progress very slowly, at both the provincial and national levels. Paradoxically, although money is said to be the greatest obstacle to achieving a capacity for health information management, in fact the biggest single roadblock, at least in Ontario, is the lack of leadership in the process of change.

PRIMARY HEALTH CARE

While it was developing its information management strategy, the commission also set about designing an approach to primary health care. The driver behind work in this area was the HSRC's recognition of primary health care as the control point, the "gateway." Reform at this first point of contact between the consumer and the health care system is critical to the objectives of continuity of care and an integrated *system* of health services. The commission believed strongly that an effective system of primary health care would play a major if not determining role in keeping people healthy — diagnosing and treating their illnesses, advocating for their care and smoothing their connection with the system when they needed in-patient care, specialist care, community care or any other health service.

Given the commission's time frame,[16] this was an ambitious goal. Several commissioners (including the chair) were of the opinion that had there been a choice at the beginning, primary health care reform/renewal might have claimed first order of priority. But by 1998 that was water under the bridge.

Faced with what appeared to be several different understandings regarding the range and scope of primary health care — and regarding its actual meaning — the HSRC established its own working definition:

> The first level of care and usually the first point of contact that people have with the health care system. Primary health care

supports individuals and families to make the best decisions for their health. It includes advice on health promotion and disease prevention, assessments of one's health, diagnosis and treatment of episodic and chronic conditions, and supportive and rehabilitative care.

[Primary health care] services are coordinated, accessible to all consumers, and are provided by health care professionals who have the right skills to meet the needs of individuals and the communities being served. These professionals work in partnership with consumers, and facilitate their use of other health-related services, when required. (HSRC 1999c)

Primary health care had been the subject of much study and debate in Ontario for decades. Prior to 1995 a number of reports had addressed a wide spectrum of issues — the principles of primary health care, funding options and potential alternative delivery models. In 1996 the Provincial Coordinating Committee on Community and Academic Health Science Centre Relations[17] had reviewed all these reports and developed recommendations on future directions for primary health care in Ontario (PCCCAR 1995a). Shortly thereafter the Ontario Medical Association's Advisory Group on Primary Care Reform (1996) (Ontario Medical Association 1996) and the Primary Care Implementation Steering Committee (1997), appointed by the Ministry of Health, addressed the same topic. In 1999 the Ontario College of Family Physicians released its own model of primary-care reform (Ontario College of Family Physicians 1999).

The commission thoroughly reviewed all of these reports with their often mutually reinforcing yet conflicting recommendations. One conclusion they all shared was that a coordinated system of primary health care had to be developed and had to be integrated with other levels of health care, including community-based and specialty services. Common themes included registering the population with groups of providers; making use of a range of health professionals; broadening the spectrum of primary-care services provided; making care available 24 hours a day, 7 days a week; motivating caregivers to broaden their range of services; adopting funding mechanisms other than fee-for-service; assuming responsibility and creating processes for the coordination of care; identifying methods and systems for quality improvement; and using information and communication technology to transform the health care system and facilitate continuous quality improvement.

The HSRC also looked at Ontario's experience with its 57 Community Health Centres (CHCs) and 77 Health Service Organizations (HSOs). CHCs were first formed in the 1960s. Their focus is the social determinants of health and health promotion and maintenance in specific hard-to-serve groups such as youths, seniors, Aboriginal people and francophones as well as homeless, transient and immigrant groups. Their salaried physicians, nurse practitioners, nurses and other health professionals work as a team to provide traditional and nontraditional primary and other services. They are funded by the Ministry of Health through global budgets. HSOs are group practices developed in Ontario in the 1970s in which patients are formally registered, or "rostered."[18] They are funded in large part by capitation payments from the Ministry of Health based on the number of people who seek primary care exclusively from the group with which they are registered. Some 10 percent of Ontario's general and family physicians practise in either CHCs (6 percent) or HSOs (4 percent).

For all the studies, debate and apparent agreement (on paper, at least) going back some 25 years on the need for change in the primary health sector and its components, little progress had been made in changing the delivery of services in Ontario. Stimulated mainly by the complaints of physicians about the patterns of their practice, the Ministry of Health and the Ontario Medical Association (OMA) had embarked jointly on some pilot reforms of primary care. However, their doctor-centred model of group practice retained fee-for-service as the basis for remuneration of physicians and blocked the introduction of nurse practitioners and other health professionals as coproviders of health care. Implementation of the pilot reforms was very slow, involved a relatively small number of physicians and was confined to certain geographical areas. The reforms were too few in number and had not been in place long enough to produce any evidence useful to the commission's study of primary health care.

When developing its own model of primary health care, the commission held round-table discussions with representatives of a number of provider groups, including the Ontario College of Family Physicians (OCFP) and the Registered Nurses Association of Ontario (RNAO). It was fully aware that the support of these groups would be critical to the successful adoption of any new model. All participants in the discussions, but particularly the OCFP and RNAO representatives, willingly shared their views with the commission, which, in turn, incorporated many of their suggestions into the model it recommended to the minister of health in November 1999 (HSRC 1999c).

During the development phase of this key report, the staff of the Ministry of Health was eerily silent, even less willing than usual to share any information — in this case about their own plans for primary care. It then became clear that their stony silence was influenced, at least in part, by the bureaucrats' behind-the-scenes discussions with OMA representatives, with whom they had been engaged in triennial negotiations over the amount of money to be added to the fee-for-service pool to provide all Ontario physicians with incremental raises. The OMA was privately if not publicly opposed even to considering any deviation from the (narrow) scope of their joint pilot initiative with the ministry. In this it was quite at odds with the OCFP over two key issues: the inclusion of nurse practitioners and other health professionals as core members of a primary-care practice, and the substitution of enrolment-based capitation payments for fee-for-service billing as the main source of physician funding. The staff of the ministry obviously had decided it was in their best interest not to rock that particular boat and to stay well away from the commission, with its propensity for boat rocking.

The commission's final report on primary health care set out clearly the organization and fundamental principles of primary health care, providing the foundation for an integrated system. The commission's model incorporated most of the elements advocated in the many existing provincial reports:

> access to a range of primary-care services, including
- health assessment
- illness prevention and health promotion
- education and support for self-care
- diagnosis and treatment of episodic and chronic illness and injuries
- primary reproductive care, including deliveries
- palliative care
- primary mental health care
- coordination and provision of rehabilitation services
- coordination of and referral to other health services such as specialist services, home care and long-term care
- supportive care in hospital, at home and in long-term-care facilities
- access to services 24 hours a day, 7 days a week, including telephone triage

> integrated group practice with a shared system of health records providing consumers with access to care and continuity of care when their customary provider (physician or nurse practitioner) is not available

> registration of consumers with their choice of primary-care physician or nurse practitioner in a group practice providing all their primary-care needs (apart from when travelling or when injured in a traffic accident or a similar emergency)
> interprofessional group practices comprising physicians, nurse practitioners and any other health professionals to meet the needs of their consumers

The commission's model differed from the others, however, in one respect — it incorporated nurse practitioners as key providers of primary health care, different from but equal to physicians in their roles as core members of Primary Care Groups, or PCGs. This was a new concept in Canada. Having conducted a thorough analysis of the administrative (billing) data available and compared them with the knowledge and skill sets required for the certification and licensure of nurse practitioners, the HSRC recognized the potential for nurse practitioners (and others with advanced training) to contribute their clinical knowledge and skills independently to the primary-care team and thereby increase its productivity. The analysis revealed that as much as 69 percent of the fee-for-service billings of primary-care physicians ($1.2 billion)[19] were for services[20] well within the competency and scope of practice of nurse practitioners.[21]

The commission was convinced that application of its PCG model could greatly improve access to primary care throughout Ontario, particularly in rural and remote communities, and could offer physicians relief from overwork, burnout and excessive on-call duty in communities with limited access to their services. The HSRC made it clear that nurse practitioners and other health professionals were not conceived, in its model, as physician substitutes or assistants; they would have the professional status of interdependent members of the PCG, with matching responsibilities, bringing to the team their own competencies and approaches to the many and varied health problems presented by patients and their families.

It came as no surprise when the model was immediately challenged by some physician groups. They claimed that, if the model were adopted, rural and remote populations would be served by PCGs with a higher proportion of nurse practitioners than urban PCGs and therefore would be subject to second-class care.[22] Interestingly, there was little reference in those criticisms to the fact that an increasing number of not so rural and remote communities were experiencing shrinking access to good primary care. As one wag remarked, sardonically, "It appears the kings of the hill don't want to share even the vacant hilltop!"

To allow for implementation of the HSRC model, a number of problems would have to be resolved, not least the fact that there were far too few nurse practitioners in Ontario to partner with family physicians in PCGs. Although education programs to qualify nurse practitioners had been in place for some time, enrolments had remained small, chiefly because of the limited employment/ practice opportunities for nurse practitioners (mainly as assistants to physicians). Therefore, along with the release of its *Primary Health Care Strategy* the commission advocated for an immediate increase in the funding of education and training for nurse practitioners (as well as midwives), to ensure an adequate supply.

The commission identified three other factors critical to the implementation and success of the PCG model:

> One or more champions had to be identified to provide leadership and assume responsibility for ensuring that renewal of primary health care received high priority both by government and by consumer and provider groups. The government responded by appointing Dr. Ruth Wilson, previously head of family medicine at Queen's University, as director of the Family Health Network, an implementation agency with its own board of directors. Following negotiations with the OMA, however, the agency's mandate was pared down considerably from what the HSRC had proposed. Also, it was placed under the firm control of the Ministry of Health's bureaucratic machinery and was not provided with the authority, flexibility or resources to foster creation of the PCG model advocated by the commission.

> Investments had to be made in the structure — mainly a governing body[23] with resources to match its responsibilities — to allow it to implement, support (financially and with human resources) and monitor change. The board of directors of the Family Health Network comprised consumer representatives, health professionals and managers, as recommended by the commission, but its mandate was restricted to the formation of group practices composed only of physicians — far from what the commission had in mind.

> The arm's-length governing body was to begin by developing a plan of action to implement reform, or "renewal," of primary health care over a six-year period. One year was to be dedicated to planning and five to implementation, with priority given to the development of PCGs in underserved areas and the conversion of group practices into PCGs.

Conversion would not be a matter of choice. The commission's analysis demonstrated that if it were voluntary, the continuation of side-by-side PCGs and fee-for-service practices, both funded under Medicare, would not be feasible from either a financial or a public service perspective. It suggested that physicians who were completely opposed to change could continue with their fee-for-service or other practice arrangements but on a private basis, outside the province's publicly funded health-insurance program.

From the beginning the commission was under no illusion that the transformation of primary care from the dominant physician-run, small-business model to its PCG model would be smooth sailing. It anticipated stiff resistance from many in the medical profession despite receiving support from the OCFP and from beleaguered practitioners working solo or in very small groups in small cities and towns and in rural and remote areas. The HSRC expected the government to be cool to the prospect of facing resistance from doctors and from organized medicine, with its ability to generate media attention and mobilize public opinion.

The commission knew full well that if its model for renewal of primary health care was to have any chance of being implemented, the case for it would have to be bolstered by compelling evidence that it did indeed represent change for the better. From the point of view of both government and potential opponents, financial considerations would be paramount. How much would conversion cost? Where would the money come from? How much better off would primary-care physicians be in terms of income, working conditions and long-term security?

Accordingly, the commission embarked on an in-depth study of the potential costs and savings of reorienting health care, putting primary care as it would be provided by PCGs at the core. After conducting a request-for-proposal process, it selected a consulting firm with an international reputation based on long experience in both health care costing and primary-care delivery.[24] (Only one Canadian company had attended a meeting of prospective bidders, and it decided not to submit a proposal because its principals thought the project "too political.")

The costing model for Inter-professional Primary Health Care Groups was based on the following assumptions:

> True group practice would be the exclusive model[25] for providers of primary health care in Ontario (replacing solo practice and/or shared practice facilities).

> The participation and role of primary health care nurse practitioners would be expanded considerably.
> A full complement of interprofessional providers would be incorporated into group practices.
> All Ontario residents would be registered with a primary-care provider within a group practice.
> Population-based funding would be the method used to pay for most primary-care services provided by the members of PCGs.

Three models of interprofessional PCGs were developed, each with its own infrastructure and staffing requirements: an *urban* model, a *rural* model and a *remote* model. The report included calculations of capitation rates appropriate for each model based on the different populations each would serve (HSRC 1999d). It also included preliminary estimates of the savings to be derived from diminution in the demand for the services of hospitals, specialists and other providers resulting from the increased capacity of PCGs to provide a comprehensive range of services.

As the commission's study proceeded throughout the spring and summer of 1999, a number of facts became clear, reinforcing its conviction that primary-care renewal would improve the system not only for consumers but also for physicians and other providers. Also, the data showed that implementation of the model would be affordable.

First, with respect to the availability of health human resources, while there were not enough nurse practitioners in Ontario to implement the HSRC model, there were enough family physicians to meet the need for those primary-care services that require their level of training and expertise; as noted previously, fully 69 percent of the total amount ($1.2 billion) billed by primary-care physicians in Ontario in 1996-97 was for services well within the scope of practice of nurse practitioners (CIHI 2003, chap. 3). In 1997-98 there were 7.9 active general/family physicians per 10,000 population (Chan 1999) and many other physicians, such as pediatricians, obstetricians, psychiatrists and internists, who provided primary care. The problem was that they were not evenly distributed between the big cities (where there were more per unit population) and less populous parts of the province. Under the commission's model, some physicians would have to relocate to small towns and rural and remote areas.

Second, allowing for a humane work week (including on-call hours) and for adequate vacation, maternity, sick and educational leave, and using the observed average of 3.22 visits to a primary-care provider per resident per year, the model allowed an average of 18 minutes of personal contact, per visit, between a consumer and his or her primary-care physician or nurse practitioner. It would put an end to the "revolving door" practices often complained about by overworked physicians and their patients. The model was based on provider:consumer ratios from 1,680 in urban areas to 1,142 in remote areas where the population was thinly distributed and harder to serve — ratios considerably smaller than those that apply now in Ontario and nationally.[26]

Third, recognizing the importance of motivating people to change and of making the new model function well, the commission costed into the model generous levels of recompense and benefits for members of the PCG team. All health professionals had to be assured that their incomes would be sustained and their working conditions improved substantially by their joining the PCGs.

Finally, with regard to affordability the commission analyzed the potential impact of a comprehensive range of primary-care services provided by PCGs on the demand for specialist services in Ontario. It concluded that demand would decrease by approximately 21 percent and that the model would generate savings approaching $1.4 billion annually. It also forecast reductions in demand in the order of 30 to 35 percent for hospital in-patient services and 15 to 20 percent for outpatient services. In total, the amount of money freed up from the diminished workload in these costly sectors would comfortably meet the costs of the six-year transition to the new model.

Throughout the intensive process of developing the *Primary Health Care Strategy*, there was strong support for primary health care as the foundation for change — as *the* means for ensuring continuity of patient care and effective utilization of services and resources across all sectors of the system envisaged by the commission.

The report was very well received (even described as a "masterpiece") and for a brief time the commission entertained the hope that some changes would be made at last. But that hope faded quickly. Behind-the-scenes resistance by vested interests and some by the public, combined with a lack of political will on the part of the government to confront the influence of organized medicine, ate away at the momentum. The model was eventually reduced to the pale shadow that was handed over in 2001, after the commission's sunset, to Ruth Wilson and the Ontario Family Health Network.

It is obvious that the medical profession's tight hold on political control of publicly funded health care will not be easily relaxed. Clearly it is not the health care consumer who is at the centre of Ontario's constellation of medical services, especially primary care.

IMPROVING HEALTH SYSTEM PERFORMANCE THROUGH GREATER ACCOUNTABILITY

In its final report on the state of Canada's health care system, the Standing Senate Committee on Social Affairs, Science and Technology (2002b), chaired by Michael Kirby, devoted part I of its discussion to accountability. The Senate Committee and Royal Commissioner Roy Romanow (Royal Commission on the Future of Health Care in Canada 2002) both recommended that priority be given to two key initiatives:

> developing the capacity to collect, share and manage health information — a precondition for measuring the performance of individual constituents (hospitals, primary health care, etc.) and the system itself

> establishing an independent National Health Council to address accountability and a vital but long-neglected question: Are we getting our money's worth?

Ontario's HSRC was a forerunner of the Kirby Committee and the Romanow Commission. One of its phase II initiatives culminated in its recommending, in March 2000, that the Ontario government develop a strategy to evaluate the performance of the system and its many components (HSRC 2000d). That strategy included the establishment of an independent, arm's-length council to approach the question from the perspective of the system as opposed to its parts. It was the commission's firm opinion that improvement of the health care system rests on a comprehensive approach to measuring its performance, identifying weaknesses and positioning it to meet future challenges.

A number of systems for monitoring and evaluating the performance of health services in Ontario had already been set up. Most noteworthy was the Institute for Clinical Evaluative Sciences (ICES), a uniquely Canadian initiative that had made great progress using secondary data in administrative databases to analyze variations in clinical practices and producing atlases that demonstrated wide regional variations.[27] However, the work of ICES was largely confined to analysis of available data; once these were distributed and made public, nobody was responsible for ensuring that the changes were made or for tracking changes and assessing the results. An initiative started by the University of Toronto and the Academic Health Science Centres was a balanced scorecard for sharing information and evaluating the performance of the five academic centres. This project was eventually taken on, and expanded to cover more hospitals, as a joint venture of the Ontario Hospital Association (OHA) and the Ministry of Health; it became known as the Hospital Report Card Project. The commission reviewed a number of similar projects initiated by a variety of organizations — the Ontario Health Regulatory Colleges, CCACs, the Toronto District Health Council and, on a national basis, CIHI and the Canadian Council on Health Services Accreditation.

Although all of these initiatives were important in evaluating the performance of particular professional groups, organizations, sectors, communities, outcomes of procedures and clinical conditions, neither the initiatives themselves nor their results were additive. In other words, they could not simply be combined and used to identify needed improvements in the performance of the health care system itself. This would require an integrated view of the system as a whole. In identifying the challenge of gaining such an integrated view, the commission noted that

> assessing health system performance assumes that there is a system to be assessed...elements that interact with one another. The notion of a system emphasizes connections and interdependencies where the whole is greater than the sum of the parts. Ontario has an extensive range of dedicated health care organizations and providers who function quite independently of each other...the interdependency and interaction that characterize a system are in [their] infancy. (HSRC 2000d)

The consultation held between the commission and the four deputy ministers of health had focused partly on how to develop a strategy for measuring and monitoring performance province-wide. The conclusion was that the first step was to partition the province into regions (as had been done in the other nine provinces), for which system-level data could then be collected and made available. But the commission found such partitioning to be a difficult task, primarily because Ontario, unlike the other provinces, has no agreed-upon regional boundaries. What it has are several different approaches to partitioning the province into geographic regions based on boundaries established by such disparate groups as the OHA, District Health Councils and Public Health Units.[28] At the time even the Ministry of Health had two sets of regions, one it had used for many years for planning purposes, and a newer set of seven regions with different boundaries established in 2000 as a result of its move to decentralize administrative functions.

At the conclusion of its study of ways and means of improving the performance and accountability of the health care system, the commission made three key recommendations:

> that the only effective approach is to focus on the system as a whole and on the *linkages* between its components or contributors (rather than on the components or contributors themselves), be they individual professional groups, institutions or health care organizations

> that an arm's-length Health System Improvement Council be set up and charged with measuring, monitoring, assessing and improving the performance of the health care system

> that consistent regional boundaries, transparent standards of information and performance benchmarks be established and publicized widely

As with the HSRC's other policy reports, its *Strategy for Improving Health System Performance* was received with great enthusiasm by many of the system's key players. But the commission was in the last months of its mandate, its influence had waned and the Ministry of Health seemed exhausted, lacking the interest and energy to consider anything new. Members of the ministry's staff freely admitted confidentially that setting up a performance monitoring system could result in the production of data that might "make the government/politicians look bad, an outcome that would, therefore, reflect poorly on the work of the bureaucracy." In the absence of strong external pressure for action (despite the complimentary rhetoric), it was easier for them to let the project wither on the shelf.

INTEGRATING THE SYSTEM FROM THE GROUND UP

Notwithstanding its observation that Ontario's health care system had yet to be created, the commission found that many throughout the province shared its conviction that working together beat working separately — that the promise of a genuine system was worth pursuing. The HSRC identified a number of local, district and regional initiatives, all centred on "champions" — volunteers and others prepared to devote time and energy to fostering cooperation and eventually integration among the various providers of health services. The goal in every initiative was to meet the needs of the population better. The approaches ranged from the specific (such as an integrated approach for children with learning and behavioural problems in

Timmins) to the general (such as a coordinated stroke strategy by the Heart and Stroke Foundation of Ontario).

Although the commission appreciated the fact that province-wide system building would require substantial "pull" from the top by the Ontario government, it also realized that a great deal could be accomplished "bottom up" by people and organizations committed to combining their resources and "pushing" together for a common purpose. Accordingly, a fourth project in phase II was an examination of ongoing initiatives in a number of communities to achieve vertical integration of health care providers. All the initiatives had been started voluntarily, the motive in every case being to bring together community players from within and outside the health care sector in order to integrate services and thereby prevent patients and their families from falling through the cracks and to increase continuity of care for vulnerable people.

The goal of the commission was to encourage these initiatives, accelerate their progress and identify (and if possible eliminate) the roadblocks to their realization. Although by then it had very few resources available for this purpose, the HSRC even distributed a few dollars to support these efforts.

Each community with an integration project was asked to develop a work plan outlining the target issue or area of its integrated effort at the local, district or regional level and how it intended to generate that effort. The commission had to be convinced that the project would lead directly to a more integrated system of care delivery. Communities were required to submit progress reports and to submit a final report by February 2000.

In its final report the commission described five very different community-based examples of what could be done by the grass roots (HSRC 2000a). It concluded, however, that without outside support and some facilitation by the Ministry of Health, such projects would have difficulty surviving. Most were reliant on a single individual to provide the continuity and energy to keep others motivated and focused. The commission foresaw that, without assistance, encouragement and an overarching policy of support for integration of the health care system at the provincial level, the vast majority of these projects would founder as the enthusiasm of their initiators waned in the face of community resistance and lack of support from the centre. As for the roadblocks, one was the fact that the ministry itself was organized into distinct program management streams, reinforced by different pieces of legislation and their associated regulations and funding streams bearing separately on hospitals, home care, physician services and so on — a different set of rules and regulation for each silo. After four years of close observation, the commission knew that few ministry personnel were inclined to change that organizational design in any significant way.

Nevertheless, as the commission completed its mandate and folded its tent, it recommended that the ministry identify someone from within its ranks to champion community-based integration projects and set up a grants program to provide seed money and support pilot projects initiated by the grass roots. This recommendation, too, was destined for the dusty shelf.

ACADEMIC HEALTH SCIENCE CENTRES

The last of the commission's phase II policy initiatives, system building, originated in its vision statement — in the concept that some of Ontario's IHSs would have particular responsibilities for the education of future physicians and other health professionals and the conduct of health research and development. Referred to as Integrated Academic Health Systems (IAHSs), they would also carry prime responsibility for the provision of highly specialized tertiary and quaternary clinical services. A fourth responsibility seen by the commission as essential was that of leadership in change — in creating partnerships and demonstrating and helping others to anticipate and meet the challenges of changing times and needs.

Its study of Ontario's five Academic Health Science Centres — in Ottawa, Kingston, Toronto, Hamilton and London — began very late in the commission's mandate and was barely a work in progress when it was truncated by the HSRC's sunset in March 2000. It built on previous work that envisaged evolution of the five centres into regional academic health-science networks incorporating many players in addition to the founding universities and teaching hospitals — community hospitals, health units, long-term-care organizations and institutions, a wide spectrum of health care providers and community-service organizations (PCCCAR 1995b). A second study provided a comprehensive review of the issues related to health human resource planning and funding for education and research (PCCCAR 1997).

Why has this good idea not been acted on? The answer to this question, the commission discovered, was much the same as the reason why the bottom-up integration projects had failed — wrecked on the shoals of indifference or opposition at the centre, most of them represented by the silo-reinforcing attitude and organization of the Ministry of Health. A contributing factor was the Academic Health Science Centres' decade-long preoccupation with financial constraints and the need to look inward for ways and means of meeting their payrolls and preserving the accessibility and quality of their services.

As it departed the scene, the commission recommended to the ministry and the five Academic Health Science Centres that together they capitalize on the potential and form Academic Health Science *Networks*; the centres would work from the bottom up in the regions and the ministry top down from the centre. Although no mechanism or champion has been found at the centre, some effective networks have been developed in the regions in which Academic Health Science Centres are located. But further progress has been slow.

Appendix 4
POLICY FORUM WORKSHOP PARTICIPANTS

Dr. Keith Banting, director of the School of Policy Studies and Dunning-Stauffer Professor of Social Policy at Queen's University (workshop chair)

Dr. John Myles, professor at Florida State University and a research fellow at Statistics Canada

Dr. Antonia Maioni, Department of Political Science at McGill University

Jacob Hacker, senior fellow at the New America Foundation and at the Brookings Institution

Dr. Carolyn Tuohy, deputy provost at the University of Toronto

Dr. Kieke Okma, senior policy adviser in the Ministry of Health, Welfare and Sport, the Netherlands

Dr. George Perlin, director of the Centre for the Study of Democracy at Queen's University

Hugh Segal, adjunct professor of public policy at the Queen's University School of Business

Present for the HSRC at the workshop were Duncan Sinclair, chair, and Beverly Nickoloff, corporate secretary

Note: Positions listed are those that applied at the time of the policy forum.

NOTES

1. Subsequently changed to recommendations when the commission's power to issue *Directions* was removed by the government, as described in chapter 4.
2. Hamilton, Kingston, London, Ottawa, Sudbury, Thunder Bay, Toronto/GTA and Windsor.
3. See chapter 8.
4. Martin Barkin, Michael Decter, Margaret Mottershead and Graham Scott. The meeting was held in July 1999.
5. The task force was chaired by Dr. Michael Guerriere, chief operating officer of the Toronto Hospital.
6. "Academic" in the sense of impractical, irrelevant, of little consequence to the "real world."
7. At least nominal. In Premier Harris's very centralized government, the premier and Management Board controlled decision-making in every ministry, the treasury possibly excepted, down to what outsiders like the HSRC considered a ridiculous level of detail.
8. Question: How many doctors does it take to change a light bulb. Answer: Change?
9. The meeting was held on April 9, 1999.
10. The parallel-path approach falls between incremental change and sweeping reform. It allows an opportunity for providers and consumers to try out alternative approaches to delivering care without dismantling or destabilizing the existing system. Since participation is optional, resistance and conflict may be reduced. Incentives are provided to encourage participation in parallel projects. There is provision for educating stakeholders on the perceived benefits of alternative delivery models and an opportunity to assess whether objectives are met.
11. Modelled, for example, on Ontario's District Health Councils.
12. Listed in very rough order of priority.
13. Information Management Working Group.
14. Then Jeff Lozon.
15. Martin Barkin, Michael Decter, Margaret Mottershead and Graham Scott.
16. Less than two years remained by then.
17. A body set up by the Ministry of Health to interface primarily with Ontario's five Academic Health Science Centres.
18. The average HSO includes three physicians.
19. In 1996-97.
20. Intermediate assessments/well-baby care, general assessments, minor assessments, individual psychotherapy and counselling.
21. *Regulated Health Professions Act*, 1991 (S.O. 1991, c. 18).
22. The ratio of physicians to nurse practitioners recommended in urban PCGs was 3:1, whereas in rural/remote PCGs it was 1:3.
23. The HSRC referred to this as an Implementation and Monitoring Committee.
24. Milliman and Robertson, Inc., Actuaries and Consultants, New York and Montreal.
25. Paid for under medicare.
26. A recent study in New Brunswick found that 45 percent of physicians between 41 and 55 years of age have practices that serve between 2,500 and 4,500 patients, and that the same proportion under 40 years of age have 1,000 to 2,500 patients. Nearly 50 percent of those under 40 were reported to be very interested in joining interdisciplinary practice teams ("Concern" 2004).
27. Established in 1992, ICES is an independent not-for-profit organization that conducts research on a broad range of topical issues to enhance the effectiveness of health care for Ontarians. Internationally recognized for its innovative use of population-based health information, ICES research provides evidence to support health-policy development and changes to the organization and delivery of health services.
28. Fourteen Local Health Integration Networks (LHIBs), with boundaries related roughly to referral patterns to tertiary care hospitals, were established in the spring of 2005.

CHAPTER 7

THE PUBLIC RELATIONS CHALLENGE

If you are contemplating change, you would be well advised to explain to those potentially affected what you have in mind, listen to what they have to say about it and then decide what to do — and when doing it, communicate, communicate, communicate. This proved to be especially true for the HSRC in 1996 as it contemplated changes to the icon that health and hospital care have become in Canada.

Early on in its mandate the commission sought the counsel of a number of people with expertise and experience in communicating with the public and reading the public's mind. To illustrate the HSRC's challenge, one such expert told the apocryphal story of a man with a very expensive wristwatch, a status symbol he looked at several times an hour.[1] Walking one day in an upscale shopping district, he was shocked to find that his watch had stopped. Happily, the shop window in front of him featured an attractive display of watches and clocks. He went in and asked the white-coated shopkeeper how long it would take to have his watch repaired. Surprised and puzzled when the shopkeeper told him they did not repair watches, the man asked what business the shop was in. Nonplussed when told that it was neutering animals, he asked, "Why, then, do you have that display of watches and clocks in your window?" The shopkeeper replied, "If you were in our line of work what would you put in the window?"

The commission's communications strategy, its "display window," had to attract public attention. The HSRC certainly did not want to mislead people about its reformist role. At the same time, it did not want to be cast as the scourge of Ontario's public hospitals, reducing their cost in order to "save the government's money." Developing the right communications/public relations strategy was essential. But this was a difficult proposition, made more so by media hype in early 1996 about the "Bully Bill" — the bill under which the HSRC had been created — and high anxiety on the part of the Ontario Hospital Association (OHA) and its member hospitals about the motives and future actions of this powerful new player. The HSRC had to not only make a positive case for hospital restructuring, but grapple with some of the negative public perceptions in evidence at the time, mainly that everything was being cut back.

In the absence of a big picture, the public had no idea why hospital restructuring was being undertaken or what a restructured system — a seamless, integrated system — might look like. In many communities, following on the work of District Health Councils (DHCs) in developing their reports on hospital restructuring, the battle lines were drawn, leaving little ground available for objective neutrality and potentially casting the HSRC as the decision-maker between winners and losers. Intensifying the generalized fear of and resistance to change were concerns among hospital unions and health care workers about labour-force adjustments and job losses. The commission's announced short time frame for implementing complex change was also a concern. The media were full of bad news, reinforcing the perception that the sole purpose of the changes to the health care system was to save money, which would mean fewer services and longer waiting lists. The headlines screamed "Tories Slashing Hospitals without Thought";[2] "Stop the 'Angel of Death' before Health Care Is Ruined";[3] "Pembroke Hospital Dispute Opens Sectarian Wounds";[4] "One Tough Job — Duncan Sinclair Is Spending the Next Four Years Shaking Up Ontario's 216 Hospitals."[5] The gloomy environment was as great a challenge as selling the commission's messages that the purpose of restructuring was to make health care better, not worse, and that it would base its decisions solely on the facts and not be influenced by newspaper headlines, emotional arguments or parochial interests.

The commission knew, its legislated power notwithstanding, that at the end of the day very little could be accomplished in the face of determined, persistent opposition from the public and, to a lesser degree, health-service providers. Accordingly, the early development of a public relations strategy claimed high priority.

One of the prime objectives was to avoid mixed messages; what was displayed in the commission's "window" had to reflect both its potential products and the processes it would use to produce them. This decision to adhere strictly to "truth in advertising" was an easy one. High on the priority list was the need for the commission to determine its core messages and then stick to them. The three criteria — quality, accessibility and affordability — constituted the kernel, closely surrounded, like cruisers around a battleship, by several others that were articulated in the early days of the commission's mandate and upheld throughout:

> The status quo is no more; it cannot and should not be preserved.
> The commission will use local planning processes (primarily those employed by the DHCs) as its starting point but will also ensure that its decisions meet what it perceives to be the evolving needs of Ontarians (e.g., aging, population growth) and take into consideration desirable changes in the patterns and practices of health care delivery.
> The commission's goal is to build a better health care system. Its mandate is not to cut costs but to find ways of preserving high-quality and accessible health services — in particular, ways of helping hospitals to deliver high-quality services despite substantial cuts to their budgets.
> The commission will reinforce the government's policy decision that all money saved through hospital restructuring be reinvested elsewhere in the health sector. Spending from the public purse on health services will be sustained[6] and not reduced over the government's four-year term.
> The commission's concern is the preservation, enhancement and affordability of health services, not the preservation of beds and buildings — or bricks and mortar.
> The commission is an independent, nonpartisan body at arm's length from government. It will work with local hospitals, DHCs and key stakeholders to ensure that hospital restructuring initiatives are appropriate both to the community concerned and to Ontario's current health and fiscal realities.

Also on the priority list was development of the capacity to deliver the message, or a communications strategy. This was not going to be easy. The commissioners and senior staff had little experience handling the media or communicating with the public in other ways.

A public relations consultant[7] was engaged to complement the succession of in-house experts[8] hired by the commission to provide advice and assist with development and implementation of a communications strategy, in order to:

> communicate the commission's decisions and messages clearly to the media, health care providers and the public
> instill confidence that the processes by which the commission received and considered information bearing on its decisions were fair, open, disciplined and effective

> explain the need for hospital restructuring in the near term and the creation of a genuine health care system in the long term, and the tangible benefits for patients and taxpayers alike
> build support throughout Ontario for the commission's decisions, recommendations and actions

The commission was keenly aware of the fact that the issue of health care has more emotional than intellectual appeal. It was aware of the profound and lasting impact of media stories about, for example, somebody's long wait for an MRI scan or a hip replacement, or having to lie for days on a gurney in a corridor waiting for an acute-care bed. The commission knew full well that when engaged in public debate it would start in a "hole," facing opposition groups armed with emotive anecdotes and well-rehearsed rhetoric of the dying-in-the-streets variety. Rejecting as fruitless the approach of trying to counter bad-news stories with good-news ones (notwithstanding the prevalence of the latter), the commission decided that its approach in communicating with both providers and the public would be to marshal and report evidence derived from objective analyses of pertinent data. Given the well-documented imbalance in public trust between politicians and health care providers (particularly family physicians and nurses), the commission also decided to stress its role as an independent, expert, impartial body, immune to lobbying. It had to counter the media's frequent references to it as the "Harris Commission" or the "Hospital Restructuring Commission." The communications strategy would address ways and means of identifying the HSRC as a body of volunteer citizens, free from political influence and interference, with an agenda that extended well beyond hospitals to all elements of health care.

The communications strategy finally adopted was simple and straightforward: stick to the core messages and communicate directly with the public and opinion leaders, through the news media and other communications vehicles (e.g., editorial board meetings and interviews), as frequently as possible.

The strategy focused on the commission's objectives and the criteria it would apply to every decision: Does it improve the quality, accessibility and affordability of health services, and will it be understood by and meet the approval of people on the street? The commissioners were volunteers from around the province with absolutely nothing to gain personally from their work on the commission; they were comparable to the legendary "dollar-a-year men" who served in Ottawa during the Second World War — citizens engaged in public service for altruistic reasons. The message was that the commission brought to its task no preconceived solutions; it would be guided solely by evidence and informed opinion, which it would welcome from any source. Finally, the only interest to be protected in all of this was the public interest.

As for getting this message out to the people of Ontario, the commission decided on four approaches:

> a province-wide focus on key opinion leaders capable of reaching the public through proactive use of the print and electronic media; every opportunity would be taken to reach the public, whether directly by speaking to any group that would listen or indirectly through media releases and interviews

> a comparable proactive initiative directed at key stakeholders and opinion leaders in the community, to raise awareness of the commission and its purpose and goals prior to its announcing decisions affecting the community

> a reactive approach in which the commission promptly responds to questions and corrects any misinformation appearing in news reports, editorials or elsewhere

> direct communication with concerned members of the Ontario legislature, health-service providers (hospitals, Community Care Access Centres, etc.) and their organizations (Ontario Hospital Association, Registered Nurses Association of Ontario, Ontario Medical Association, etc.), health planners and advocacy groups (DHCs, foundations, associations, etc.) and municipal governments

The implementation plan was also straightforward. First, every attempt would be made to identify potential allies — those supportive of the commission and its goals who could help to get the message out to the public. At the top of the list were the editorial boards of newspapers, especially the Toronto dailies, and those responsible for public affairs programs on radio and television.

At the outset the HSRC underestimated the importance of dealing directly with the media. It assumed that its well-researched and well-argued reports would speak for themselves and obviate the need for the chair, chief executive officer or other spokespersons to meet with editorial boards and reporters. Such meetings, though often stressful, proved to be extraordinarily important elements in the commission's communications strategy, serving to explain to the public what it was trying to accomplish and why. The commissioners and chief executive officer treated every invitation as an opportunity for reasoned debate[9] and took advantage of every chance to communicate with the media and participate in newsworthy events. The HSRC's processes for hospital restructuring contained built-in strategies to facilitate communication with the public in every community affected. There was a call for written submissions followed by face-to-face meetings with stakeholders. Each community visit began with a local press conference. Following the release of *Notices* and *Directions*, the commissioners sought to meet with local media representatives and political leaders to address questions relating to the HSRC's decisions. Finally, a few media spokespersons were identified (the fewer the better, according to the commission's advisers).

The last involved the commissioners, the chief executive officer and some senior staff members in what proved to be a trying, frustrating, even frightening exercise — media training! After a brief but thorough education session, the HSRC's consultants brought in a highly experienced interviewer together with a technical team replete with lights, cameras, recorders, monitors and metres of cable running hither and yon. Each potential spokesperson — a rank amateur facing an aggressive, well-informed and deliberately hostile interviewer — was challenged to respond to a series of rapid-fire questions and comments designed to expose one's public demeanour and attitude and test one's ability to represent the commission under adverse conditions. Many of the questions were of the no-acceptable-answer genre ("What are you doing to repair your reputation since your conviction for tax evasion?"). After watching the replays, embarrassing to the interviewee and hilarious to everybody else, the consultants went quickly around the room and identified the small number of interviewees they thought capable, with coaching and training, of speaking for the commission. Asked how they could be so certain of their selections after such brief exposure, the experts spoke of "sticking to the core messages," "giving succinct sound bites," "quick thinking," "short answers," "absence of jargon" and "few ums and ahs," but also about what they described as the all-important reaction of the camera — "It either likes you or it doesn't." If the camera doesn't like you, the best anybody can do, even with expert makeup, media training and experience, is gain its grudging tolerance. It is a scary prospect: an age so dominated by the visual image that the potential of leadership and the power of argument are determined by an electronic or mechanical device (and its operator).

Despite this careful selection process, the commission's chair and chief executive officer, more or less by default and by virtue of their availability, went on to more intensive media coaching and, with experience (lessons under fire), became its primary spokesmen. Luckily, according to the expert consultants, the all-discerning camera liked both of them well enough from the beginning.

Throughout the commission's four-year mandate, especially in its first two years, there was no shortage of invitations to speak to gatherings of health care providers and planners and to general audiences such as members of the Canadian Club. Some groups were national in scope, the majority were provincial and a considerable number were local; audiences were small, and media coverage was modest. With its fast start on hospital restructuring, Thunder Bay was chosen by the national and provincial media, both print and electronic, as the bellwether of the commission's approach — which, of course, it was. This led to extensive reporting, most of it favourable, on how the HSRC's analytical and decision-making processes were applied and worked there, how its *Notices* were modified by the invited reactions to them, and how its final *Directions* and recommendations were received. In Sudbury, similarly, the extensive national, provincial and local coverage of the amalgamation of three competing institutions into a regional hospital on one site, including coverage of the Sisters of St. Joseph of Sault Ste. Marie's appeal to the court for a stay of the *Directions*,[10] generated a good deal of exposure and support for the commission's message.

Not everything was positive. The commission had plenty of opportunity to use the third arrow in its communications quiver — that of reacting promptly to misinformation and queries. But on the whole, from very early on the HSRC was satisfied with the effectiveness of its communications strategy in transmitting its messages to the public and communicating directly with health care providers and others. The constant challenge was to ensure that the messages and the communications process were driven by facts, not emotion or symbolism.

As for execution of the communications strategy, about a year into the life of the commission, in response to concerns about the degree of "fit" so far achieved, a new team of public relations/communications consultants[11] was engaged to advise on ways of promoting the HSRC's messages more extensively, effectively and accurately. Subsequently, in a more direct approach to communicating its decisions and the reasons for them, the HSRC began to purchase full-page advertisements in local newspapers the day after the release of its *Notices* or *Directions*. The ads invited questions and comments as well as requests for additional information. It had not proved possible to guarantee such complete and accurate information in every community when the commission relied solely on media reports for the purpose; the number, ability, comprehension and experience of reporters assigned by local media outlets to the story varied widely. The commission was persuaded that the public interest warranted the expense of purchasing advertising space, ensuring both transparency and the accurate and timely informing of people in every community affected by its decisions. In respect of the latter, on the days when its *Notices* and *Directions* were released the HSRC held formal briefings for hospital leaders and others directly affected well in advance of releasing media representatives from their "lock-up." This provided board chairs, members and chief executive officers an opportunity to communicate the commission's decisions directly to hospital employees and others. The commission usually provided reporters with embargoed copies of its reports so their stories could go to print soon after official release of its *Notices* or *Directions*. This was much appreciated by reporters, especially those covering a broad spectrum of events and topics in small communities, who were often left scrambling to get up to speed quickly on the complex issues dealt with by the HSRC. The representatives of one newspaper said, "It will improve your chances of getting a positive story if you give us an advance copy of the report and time to digest it before writing about it."

The HSRC also sharpened the tone of its messages to reveal its growing concern over the government's failure to respond to its recommendations, mainly in relation to reinvestments in home care and long-term care but also in capital investment in hospitals. It was also increasingly concerned with the system's resistance to change in the face of compelling evidence of the need for it. Accordingly it became more proactive in seeking opportunities to make its message heard, especially during the first two years of its mandate.

How effective was the commission in communicating its objectives to the public and to health care providers? It did no polling to assess the public's awareness of and reaction to its activities, but, judging from the extensive media coverage, the commission was certainly talked about. The commissioners and their professional advisers concluded that the communications strategy had been as effective as could be expected given the resources of time, personnel and money devoted to it. In the spring of 2004 feedback on the commission's effectiveness as communicator was sought from some of the Toronto reporters and columnists who had most frequently covered its activities. The consensus was that the HSRC had been open, transparent, and forthcoming and that its chair and chief executive officer had been readily available to the media. The fact that this positive assessment did not extend to the Ontario government or to the minister and the Ministry of Health is a matter beyond the commission's purview.

The commission's repeated use of its extensive mailing lists to distribute information to individual hospitals and a range of organizations representing various provider communities led it to believe that its message was being heard within the "system." It was impossible to determine, however, if it was reaching more than a small sampling of individual health professionals in this manner. There was no vehicle for communicating reliably with all doctors or all nurses in all their diversity of practice, employment, specialities and interests, much less with health professionals across the board.

The commission developed and maintained a Web site on which it posted all of its restructuring reports and discussion papers as they became available. Judging from the number of "hits" and the volume of the feedback received, this was an increasingly effective channel of communication. Subsequent to the commission's sunset, the Web site and its maintenance were transferred to the Ministry of Health. Over time it became enigmatically coded and more and more difficult to access. In the spring of 2004 the site was closed down by the ministry, but its contents are still available.[12]

Quite apart from evaluating the commission's success in reaching the general public and health care providers, it was difficult to determine the extent to which the objectives of the communications strategy were being achieved. Were people aware that the commission was functioning at arm's length from government and was focused on protecting and enhancing affordable, accessible, high-quality health care? Was the HSRC seen in a more positive light as a result of its communications strategy? Did Ontarians believe that it was genuinely acting in the public interest and that its real objective was not to save the government money? Although the commissioners were resolutely opposed to spending money to sample public opinion, they were satisfied with their positive interactions with providers and members of the public and with the responses, via media reports, letters and the Web site, to their published reports and to speeches by their chair and chief executive officer. Undoubtedly some of that positive feedback came from the converted, those who welcomed the kind of changes the commission was recommending. Even with that caveat, however, the consensus was that, in an emotionally charged area such as health care, members of the public and health care providers alike took a remarkably positive view of the HSRC.

The majority of the many speaker requests that came to the commission were filled by the chairman or the chief executive officer, but other commissioners were pressed into service from time to time, especially if the event was to be held in their home communities. Following the release of the commission's *Directions* in Windsor, however, the chairman was invited by a member of the Ontario legislature, Sandra Pupatello,[13] to meet with residents concerned about people lined up in emergency rooms waiting for a bed to become available in the hospitals being restructured. The chair, having already contacted Doug Lawson, a Windsor resident, declined, saying that a commissioner was available locally. Pupatello replied, "Oh, I couldn't do that to Doug!"

One of the frustrations in trying to enlist the support of opinion leaders in the media was the extent to which political ideology influenced editorials and commentary following HSRC interviews with editorialists and journalists. The commission's representatives were given several opportunities to present opinion leaders with evidence and arguments that had proved to be entirely convincing to other audiences. Naively confident, after a vigorous in-depth discussion, that it had made a good case, the commission was sometimes disappointed to read subsequent editorials and commentaries that were ideologically slanted by concepts, sometimes of a politically partisan nature, that had never even entered the conversation. The commissioners fully appreciated the role of editorialists and columnists as opposed to that of reporters, having been warned by their in-house experts and consultants not to expect the same degree of objectivity from the two groups: news is one thing, opinion another. They were nevertheless surprised at the degree to which ideological "capture" affected some members of the Fourth Estate, wielding their enormous power to influence and even form public opinion. They concluded that the press is not nearly as free or objective as it purports to be.

The commission made a practice of responding quickly and openly to the inquiries of journalists, especially those few assigned to the health or health-policy beat. Whenever it was on the point of releasing a report that its advisers thought might constitute a story, the HSRC set up a news conference in Toronto for issues of broad provincial interest (such as the formation of the commission itself and the division of its work into two phases), and in the communities affected when it concerned local hospital restructuring. The HSRC came to appreciate how thin on the ground experienced reporters are and the difficulties they face in gathering even minimal background information, much less the in-depth knowledge necessary to do justice to their many diverse assignments. This seemed particularly true of television and radio journalists — who had to provide sound bites for almost immediate broadcast. On the whole, however, the commission found its confidence in the competency and objectivity of journalists to be well placed. Given the extraordinary time constraints under which they worked, their reports reflected a remarkable grasp of the issues and a fair representation of both the various positions and the HSRC's objective: a genuine system of health care in Ontario.

In 1999, as the hospital-restructuring phase began to wind down, the commission turned its attention to communication of a different kind — ways and means of offering providers and the public an overview of its system-building work. In terms of the hospital sector, for example, the challenge was to use a province-wide context to illustrate to people the emotion-laden changes made to their local hospital. This required the preparation of what the commission began to call "legacy reports," documents that could be widely distributed and thus live on into the future; they could serve as a foundation for both measurement of the value of the HSRC's work to Ontario and efforts to advance the course of "reorganizing and revamping the delivery system," to quote Tommy Douglas.

The first of these legacy reports concerned hospital restructuring; it included a 15-page plain-language summary of the situation prior to phase I, common myths and facts regarding the process, the results, and a call for comments, suggestions and opinions (HSRC 1999a). It pointed out that between 1989 and 1995 (before the HSRC's arrival on the scene), 11,000 hospital beds had been closed in Ontario.[14] A large proportion of these were surgical beds, reflecting the rapid shift from in-patient to outpatient surgery. During the same period hospital funding had increased by 20 percent.[15] After completion of the HSRC restructuring of all urban hospitals (which in 2005 is still some time in the future), the total number of beds in every category except rehabilitation will be decreased yet further (under 14 percent in total, under 12 percent in acute care[16]), but the total capacity of the system will be increased by nearly 40 percent, to 375,000 beds and places, through the creation of large numbers of long-term-care beds (over 36 percent) and home-care places (over 41 percent) and a 48 percent increase in home-care capacity to accommodate patients discharged from hospital. Despite the impression left by hospitals and the media that the HSRC was further reducing acute-care capacity, implementation of the commission's *Directions* would have had the opposite effect had sufficient funds been provided through to 2003

— acute-care capacity was to be increased by facilitating patient throughput, making more effective and efficient use of hospital capacity via improved coordination between hospitals and other players in the system. Briefly put, the changes wrought by the commission were intended to increase substantially the system's ability to meet the demand for hospital and other services. All this would have been achieved at an annual reinvestment cost of $1.2 billion, two-thirds of it realized by savings of $800 million in the hospital sector. Clearly, the commission's purpose was not to save the government money! Capital reconstruction of Ontario's public hospitals, costing in the order of $2 billion, would have gone some way toward modernizing the buildings and would have permitted an 18 percent increase in emergency and ambulatory visits. The government had already committed an additional $2 billion for the construction of new long-term-care beds. The commission ordered the closure of 33 public hospital sites; most of these have closed or are in the process of doing so and many have been converted to ambulatory-care centres, nursing homes or seniors' residences. The HSRC also advised the minister to close six Provincial Psychiatric Hospitals and divest their management to community boards, and to close six private hospitals; quick action was taken on part of that advice but some has yet to be acted upon. Fourteen amalgamated urban hospitals were created from 44 separate organizations.

The commission had hoped that this report, produced mainly by its third in-house communications expert, Paul Kilbertus, would be picked up by the media as a good-news story and would reinforce the public's expectations for the more policy-oriented system-building work to come in phase II. Although it received some attention, the "good" proved once again not to fit the definition of news nearly as well as the "bad." The summary report on hospital restructuring, although useful for health-policy experts and their students, sank quickly without the public notice it deserved.

As 1999 proceeded into fall and winter, discussions with the Ontario Archives were initiated to ensure preservation of the commission's voluminous files of correspondence, reports and working papers. An agreement was reached with the Canadian Health Services Research Foundation in Ottawa on its taking over the distribution of the commission's final legacy report. As noted, the Ministry of Health agreed to maintain the Web site.

Near the end of its mandate the commission engaged the services of Margaret Mottershead, the deputy minister of health who had played such an instrumental role in its formation then retired from the public service, to draw together information for inclusion in the final legacy report the commission had decided to put on the public record before closing its doors. Mottershead conducted a series of 30 interviews with influential people within and outside of government familiar with the commission's work, as part of a "looking back, looking forward" project. The "looking back" segment dealt with the HSRC's legislated authority, mandate and processes, as well as the outcomes and an evaluation of its work. "Looking forward" comprised the interviewees' opinions on the structures and actions needed postcommission for Ontario to continue moving forward and to build, out of the "field of silos," an effective and efficient health-services system. Although the sample was small, Mottershead's report leaves no doubt that the commission and its work were well known, that its achievements were significant and that it had remained well distanced from government throughout.

This work by Mottershead was combined with the commission's thorough analysis of its own records and incorporated into *Looking Back, Looking Forward* (HSRC 2000b). This final legacy report provides an overview of the commission's approach to the restructuring of health services in the period April 1996 to March 2000 and summarizes the results of its work to that time. It provides the rationale for beginning with hospital restructuring, pointing out that phase I was intended in part to prevent the serious disruptions in service that would have resulted had Ontario's 220 public hospitals acted individually on the huge reductions imposed on their budgets beginning in 1996. It also included the results of a final study by the HSRC, a summary of workforce-adjustment policies and strategies — a health human resources report arising out of hospital restructuring. *Looking Back, Looking Forward* pointed out, however, that the commission's principal objective was to lay the foundation for a sensibly sized, rationalized, coordinated hospital sector capable of participating in, if not leading, the development of the integrated, comprehensive health-services system that was the commission's focus in phase II. It was during this latter phase that the HSRC developed the series of strategies — health information management, primary-care reform, evaluation of performance and accountability — needed to realize its vision of the seamless health-services system needed to optimize the health of Ontarians into the twenty-first century.

The legacy report and its accompanying *Seven Points for Action* (HSRC 2000c) were the principal documents released to the public by the HSRC. The former evaluated the performance of the commission against its goal of providing patients and their families with better continuity of care and taxpayers with the cost-effectiveness that results from proper coordination among providers of a wide spectrum of health care services. The report concluded that the HSRC was a necessary and effective force for change that fulfilled its mandate and discharged its responsibilities well, but that much remained to be done — hence the commission's recommended seven next steps:

(1) Build on the base established by the HSRC; complete the implementation of hospital restructuring and reinvestment in other health facilities and community services.
(2) Articulate and communicate to the public a vision of the health-services system in Ontario.
(3) Clarify and define the role of government as primarily responsible for governance, leadership and accountability throughout the health-services system.
(4) Develop a comprehensive health information management system to support the governance and management of health services throughout Ontario.
(5) Implement a new model of comprehensive primary health care.
(6) Foster and support improved coordination and integration of health care providers, first by reinforcing local community efforts and stimulating the formation of academic health science networks.
(7) Develop and implement a strategy to improve accountability for health-system performance.

When *Looking Back, Looking Forward* and *Seven Points for Action* were released in March 2000 the Health Services Restructuring Commission was old news. The doors to its office at 56 Wellesley Street West were closed, its reports and files were transferred to the Archives of Ontario, a final audit was concluded and the assets, together with any ongoing responsibilities, were handed over to the Ministry of Health. All remaining personnel returned to the departments, institutions and organizations from which they had been seconded or went on to new positions and challenges or to retirement. The commissioners hung on their study walls the framed mounts of their four dollars signed by Premier Mike Harris and his health minister, Elizabeth Witmer, and quietly went their separate ways.

Seven Points for Action, directed at the Ontario government, was, apart from a modest and very constrained start on primary-care renewal, promptly added to the ministry's no doubt lengthy "to do" list. But the commission's final legacy report, *Looking Back, Looking Forward*, has not faded away. Although increasingly dated, as all reports will be, it has somehow escaped the dusty fate of countless others by commissions, task forces and committees established to provide advice and recommendations. It continues to communicate the commission's ideas and purposes to a large and varied audience provincially, nationally and even internationally. As the HSRC closed its doors and its reports became widely available, a high degree of consistency began to emerge from Quebec's Clair Commission, Saskatchewan's Fyke Commission and Alberta's Mazankowski Health Council, all of which had been established to foster system building in their respective provinces. As we have seen, some of the same core recommendations — strong governance, improved health information management, primary-care reform — were featured more recently in reports by the Standing Senate Committee chaired by Senator Michael Kirby and by Royal Commissioner Roy Romanow.

The commission's communications strategy proved to be quite successful. Its ideas still have legs.

NOTES

1. The expert was Allan Gregg, former president of Decima Research (and now of Strategic Counsel), pollster for the federal Conservatives, broadcaster, columnist, consultant and rock band manager.
2. *Toronto Star*, October 8, 1996.
3. *Toronto Star*, May 25, 1997.
4. *Ottawa Citizen*, June 7, 1997.
5. *Toronto Star*, September 15, 1996.
6. In constant (1995) dollars, not allowing for inflation.
7. Initially Temple Scott.
8. Initially Jane Stewart (seconded from the Ministry of Health), followed by Ruth Lewkowicz (seconded from North York General Hospital) and finally Paul Kilbertus (seconded from the Ministry of Health).
9. There were some that did not meet this criterion.
10. See chapter 8.
11. Environics Communications.
12. See http://www.health.gov.on.ca/hsrc/home.htm.
13. Now minister of community and social services.
14. From 49,000 (including 33,000 acute-care beds) to 38,000 (including 24,000 acute-care beds).
15. From $6 billion in 1989 to $7.3 billion in 1995.
16. In fact, at the planning horizon of 2003 the reduction was even greater by virtue of the fact that insufficient resources were available to hospitals to achieve the bed targets set by the HSRC (see table 1 in chapter 4).

CHAPTER 8

LEGAL CHALLENGES

One of the more time-consuming and expensive aspects of the commission's work related to what its first chief executive officer, Mark Rochon, wryly called its "busy legal practice." He was referring to the several court challenges that were mounted by hospitals in response to (and, once, in anticipation of) *Directions* issued during phase I, hospital restructuring. Denied the time-honoured wielding of political influence by the commission's arm's-length relationship to the government and the premier's injunction to "stand clear," hospitals had no way to head off HSRC decisions that they believed would not serve their interests. Naturally, they adopted the only tactics remaining to them when such decisions were made. Most acquiesced and proceeded with good grace into relationships with other hospitals as they had been directed to do. But some did everything possible to mobilize public opinion against the commission's orders, hoping to create such a furor that the government would be spurred into acting on their behalf or, more likely, into foot-dragging with regard to recommendations for funding, and that the delay would make the problem go away. A third option, often combined with the second, was to appeal to the courts.

SUDBURY GENERAL

The commission's first challenge came in January 1997, when the Sisters of St. Joseph of Sault Ste. Marie, owners and operators of the Sudbury General Hospital, brought an application to the Divisional Court for judicial review of *Directions* issued in mid-December. They also moved before a judge of the court to put the *Directions* in abeyance pending the hearing of their application by a full, three-judge panel. The *Directions* called for the hospital to collaborate with two other hospitals[1] to establish, by the end of April, a new consolidated hospital corporation to which all three would transfer their assets and then cease to exist. The three together were also to collaborate with a fourth hospital,[2] which would be responsible for all hospital-based mental health services in the area. The commission had appointed two experienced facilitators, Graham Scott[3] and Maureen Quigley, to help Sudbury's four hospitals find a mutually satisfactory way of combining their efforts to meet the needs of the community and region for hospital-based services. The Sisters and representatives of the Sudbury General Hospital had agreed to participate in the process on a "without prejudice" basis pending the judicial review. The biggest single roadblock was the religious element — how to partner the Sisters' hospital with the others.

The Sisters' case against the *Directions* was that the creation of a single regional hospital was impossible unless the hospital was governed by a board controlled by the Roman Catholic Church; that their freedom of religion under the Canadian Charter of Rights and Freedoms would be infringed if they were denied the right to operate a religious hospital; and that transfer of their hospital's assets to a secular hospital ran counter to canon law. The Sisters argued that a stay should be granted to prevent any further steps toward infringement of their rights until the court had dealt fully with their claims. Before issuing its *Directions*, the commission was aware of the restrictions placed on religious institutions by canon law, a body of ecclesiastical principles and rules derived from papal and Roman Catholic Church pronouncements.[4] Early on in its mandate the HSRC had consulted a number of Canadian and international experts about the limits set by canon law on various forms of collaboration between Roman Catholic and secular hospitals. As with most laws and most experts, interpretations varied. Some experts held strictly to the view that the separateness of Catholic hospitals was absolute and inviolate under canon law, whereas others believed there was considerable room to manoeuvre. All agreed, however, that Roman Catholic hospitals could not be merged with their secular counterparts without offence to canon law.

The court[5] found that these claims did indeed raise serious issues that should be decided by a full panel of judges in the hearing of the Sisters' application for judicial review of the *Directions*, scheduled for early April, approximately 10 weeks off. However, the court rejected the request for a stay pending that hearing.

It found that the Sisters would suffer no irreparable harm in the interim. On the other hand, there was overwhelming evidence that hospital restructuring in the Sudbury area was long overdue. The public and the other hospitals would be much more inconvenienced than the Sisters if planning and other activities related to hospital restructuring were to be suspended until after the judicial review.

Subsequently the commission's confidence in facilitated negotiations was reinforced, along with its faith in the ability of people to develop amicable solutions to even the most difficult of situations. The Sisters withdrew their application for a judicial review when they accepted the role of partner with the new Sudbury Regional Hospital Corporation in developing and providing all long-term, complex continuing and palliative care at the new facility. The commission amended its *Directions* to accommodate this solution and everybody moved on. Many are entitled to a share of the credit for the success of hospital restructuring in the Sudbury region, but most of the credit belongs to the Sisters of St. Joseph of Sault Ste. Marie, for courageously and sensitively balancing their faith-based principles with the need to collaborate with their secular counterparts to better meet the needs of the population.

The only sour note emanating from this story relates to unfounded allegations of bias levelled against Commissioner George Lund, a long-time Sudbury resident previously active in the governance of the Algoma Hospital and the mental health programs of Network North. Despite incontrovertible evidence of Lund's adherence to the HSRC's conflict-of-interest guidelines, including his abstaining from all HSRC decisions relating to his community, rumour mongering continued until the win-win nature of what had been achieved dawned on even the most hidebound of opponents to change.

ONTARIO PUBLIC SERVICE EMPLOYEES UNION

The second court challenge to the commission was brought by the Ontario Public Service Employees Union (OPSEU) in April 1997, six months after the release of the HSRC's *Directions* in Thunder Bay.[6] The OPSEU asserted that Lakehead Psychiatric Hospital[7] was not defined as a public hospital under the *Public Hospitals Act* — ironically, because, like all Provincial Psychiatric Hospitals (PPHs), it was owned and operated directly by the Ontario government — and therefore was not subject to the authority of the commission.

The commission did not dispute the point. It agreed that its *Directions* bearing on that hospital had been issued in error. The HSRC had the power to advise the minister on matters relating to PPHs, but not to issue them the binding directions that applied to public hospitals under the Act. Since there was no dispute as to the commission's jurisdiction, the court dismissed the application for judicial review. In the end, however, the commission's restructuring did greatly affect Ontario's psychiatric hospitals. Shortly after the release of the HSRC's report on hospital restructuring in Thunder Bay, the minister of health notified the commission of his intention to act on its recommendations as they applied to PPHs throughout the province. The minister advised the HSRC to treat PPHs just as it was treating public hospitals but instead of issuing *Directions* to provide advice directly to him as chair of their governing body — that is, the ministry.

PEMBROKE CIVIC

Coincident with these two skirmishes in court, the commission faced its first major challenge following its review of hospital services in Renfrew County. In February 1997 it had released its final report ordering the closure of the emergency department of one of Pembroke's two public hospitals, the Civic, by the end of June — later amended to July — and the hospital itself by the end of the year. The Civic, together with one of its patients, applied in June for a stay of the order to close the emergency department pending a full judicial review. The hearing of the application was originally scheduled for November but, through the efforts of the parties, was brought forward to July. Following the precedent established in Sudbury, the court found that the "anchor" of the hospital's application — that it would suffer irreparable harm if its emergency department were to be closed prior to a full judicial review — had "entirely disappeared" because the hearing would now take place before the amended date of closure.[8] The motion to stay was dismissed.

The application was heard a month later. The decision dismissing the application, written by Mr. Justice Archie Campbell, would itself prove to be a solid anchor against challenges to the commission's power to restructure public hospitals in Ontario.[9]

One of the commissioners who participated in the Renfrew County review observed that visiting Pembroke, a handsome Ottawa Valley community, was akin to stepping back into the nineteenth century, at least with respect to the influence of religion on daily life. The city seemed to be divided, architecturally and functionally, between Roman Catholics and Protestants, bringing to mind the Blues and Buffs of Charles Dickens's Eatanswill in *The Pickwick Papers*. In this two-hospital community, the question of religious ownership was a hot topic, as evidenced by the reception to a report by the Renfrew District Health Council, which had pointed out the qualitative and financial advantages of consolidating the community's hospital services in one institution.

The commission agreed with the recommendations of the Renfrew DHC. In addition to closure of the secular Civic, it ordered expansion of the Pembroke General, a Roman Catholic hospital owned by the Grey Sisters, to accommodate all hospital-based needs of the population. Many on the secular side of the community were incensed at the prospect of having to seek care at a hospital in which crucifixes were prominently displayed and "Roman Catholicism will be shoved down our throats."

Addressing first the role of the court in reviewing the commission's decisions, Mr. Justice Campbell recognized the broad powers of the commission and the limits on the court's ability to intervene:

> The court has no power to inquire into the rights and wrongs of hospital restructuring laws or policies, the wisdom or folly of decisions to close particular hospitals, or decisions to direct particular hospital governance structures. It is not for the court to agree or disagree with the decision of the Commission. The law provides no right of appeal from the Commission to the court. The court has no power to review the merits of the Commission's decisions. The only role of the court is to decide whether the Commission acted according to law in arriving at its decision.

With respect to the Civic's claim that the HSRC had exceeded its powers by considering, as a matter of policy, preservation of denominational health care, the court found that the commission was right to consider Ontario's long tradition of diversity in hospital governance and that it had acted within its powers by doing so. The court also noted that this should not have come as a surprise given that the subject had been much discussed in the community since publication of the Renfrew DHC report, well before the commission had arrived on the scene.

The Civic also alleged procedural unfairness because the HSRC had not provided it with adequate disclosure of the case it was expected "to meet" and copies of all the submissions made by others. The court found no unfairness, given the commission's function:

> The HSRC was a policy-making and implementation body, not an adversarial forum. It was not obliged to adopt the adversarial procedures of a court or to provide production and discovery. It was obliged to give the [hospital] a fair opportunity to make its views known to the commission before it issued its directions and it did so. The language of the "case to meet" principle has great application to adversarial proceedings where there is a *lis* between two adversaries. It has much less application to a complex polycentric decision like that of the HSRC in restructuring the local health care system.

The third claim was that the commission had contravened the Charter of Rights and Freedoms because abortions and related reproductive services were not and would not be provided at the General Hospital. The court noted that no abortion had been performed in either of Pembroke's two hospitals for as long as anyone could remember. It quoted uncontested evidence by the General's chief of obstetrics and gynecology that he had never experienced any interference of a religious nature in obstetric or gynecological decisions. With respect to the applicant's concern about religious influence on patients, the court found no evidence of such influence. It also pointed out that "the silent presence of crosses and crucifixes…does not infringe any Charter religious rights" and, furthermore, that the Charter challenge was "premature and speculative"; nobody had ever complained of being denied services of any kind.

The applicants also accused the commission of closed-minded prejudgment of the case, despite the fact that the HSRC had rejected a more-or-less status quo governance proposal put forward by the General; it had ordered that the new board of governors be fully representative of the population, reflect the community's demographic, cultural, linguistic, geographic, ethnic, religious and social characteristics, and engage in a fair and equitable nomination and election process. The court noted that this demonstrated an open rather than a closed mind on the part of the commission.

The court rejected the claim of bias on the part of the commission as "particularly thin" and dismissed the application for a judicial review of its ordering the closure of the Civic's emergency department and the hospital itself. The Civic promptly applied for leave to appeal that decision. It sought and was granted[10] a temporary stay of its obligation to comply with the HSRC's *Directions* pending disposition of the application for leave to appeal. That application was dismissed in September.[11]

The emergency department and later the hospital were closed. The community, although continuing to struggle over the formation of an appropriately representative governing body, got on with restructuring the Pembroke General to play its new role as provider of hospital services for the whole community.

But as the commission's focus on hospital restructuring was expanded to encompass other communities, more legal troubles were brewing.

WELLESLEY CENTRAL HOSPITAL AND DOCTORS HOSPITAL, TORONTO

The commission's "busy legal practice" was made even busier in June 1997 with another application to the court. This time the Wellesley Central Hospital in Toronto applied for a judicial review of the HSRC's *Notices of Intention to Issue Directions*. In these *Notices*, released in early March, about midway in its very complex review of Metropolitan Toronto, the HSRC gave notice of its favouring closure of the Wellesley Central and the transfer of its programs to St. Michael's Hospital; these two hospitals would then operate a new ambulatory-care hospital on the site of the former Central Hospital, located midway between the two. The application by the Wellesley Central was dismissed on the grounds that it was premature to request a review of decisions the commission had yet to make.[12] The *Notices*, in fact, invited those potentially affected to present evidence and arguments why the commission should pursue alternative solutions.

In fact the Wellesley Central Hospital had repeatedly communicated with the HSRC during the "notice" period. Perhaps when it made its submission to the court in June it lacked sufficient confidence in its arguments to persuade the commission. In any case the *Directions* for hospital restructuring in Metropolitan Toronto, issued a month later, indicated that the HSRC had not changed its mind. Wellesley Central promptly applied for a judicial review, this time of the *Directions*. The application was heard by the court in late August and Mr. Justice O'Connor's decision dismissing the application was rendered in mid-September.[13]

Almost simultaneously, Doctors Hospital, also located in Toronto, applied for a judicial review, seeking to quash the commission's *Directions* to relocate and relinquish the operation and management of its programs to the Toronto Hospital (TTH), a teaching hospital affiliated with the University of Toronto. This application was heard by the same panel of judges who had just heard the Wellesley Central one, and the decision dismissing the Doctors Hospital case, written by Mr. Justice Southey, was released on the same mid-September day.[14]

The application by Doctors Hospital related primarily to the HSRC's jurisdiction and, therefore, the validity of its *Directions*. The claim was that it had exceeded its powers by changing the recommendation of the Metro Toronto DHC that Doctors Hospital relocate but retain "autonomous control" of its ambulatory-care centre on the premises of the Western Hospital Division of TTH. In its review of the legislative and regulatory foundations for the commission's powers, including that of acting in place of the minister of health in issuing directions under the *Public Hospitals Act*, the court found that the HSRC did "have regard" for the DHC's plan, as it was required to do, but that there were no limits to the changes it could make to that plan; it had acted within its powers.

Doctors Hospital also claimed that the commission, because it had not made specific reference to the public interest, had failed to consider the public interest in its *Directions*. Quoting directly from the HSRC's *Notice of Intention to Issue Directions*, issued in March, and from its *Directions*, issued in September, the court rejected this contention: "It is quite apparent, in my opinion, that the commission was acting in what it believed to be the public interest."

The hospital also claimed that the HSRC had exceeded its authority by considering the interests of the University of Toronto and that its conduct gave rise to apprehension of bias because it had asked Dr. Arnold Aberman, dean of medicine, and Professor Robert Prichard, president of the university, to act as facilitators in (failed) attempts to reach agreement between Doctors and TTH. It also contended an apprehension of bias in remarks by the commission's chair to the Ontario Hospital Association admitting that he was personally concerned about accommodating the needs and contributions of teaching hospitals beyond what most members of the OHA would find acceptable.

Following upon the ruling of Mr. Justice Campbell in the Pembroke Civic Hospital case, Mr. Justice Southey affirmed the breadth of the commission's authority:

> Although the Commission must consider the public interest, its powers are virtually unfettered. The Commission is the surrogate

of the Minister. Regulation 87/96 under the Public Hospitals Act provides that the Commission, in relation to the Minister's powers...to close hospitals and issue directions to the hospital administrator, may issue directions in the place of the Minister. The Commission stands in the shoes of the Minister and exercises the Minister's powers. On the spectrum between political decision-making and judicial decision-making, the Commission is close to the extreme political/legislative end of the spectrum.

In addition, the court found that the statement by the HSRC chair on which Doctors Hospital had relied "did not begin to establish" that he had a closed mind on the matters considered by the commission.

Doctors also submitted that the *Directions* would have the effect of expropriating its property, a power that had not been expressly conferred on the commission by statute. The court found that the *Directions* did not result in expropriation: they required only a change in oversight of program and services at Doctors Hospital, and TTH would have only temporary use of the buildings and assets of Doctors to facilitate the transition.

On the charge that parts of the *Directions* were vague and therefore void, the court pointed to the complexities of restructuring health care in Metropolitan Toronto and to the expectation that Doctors Hospital actively seek to convert the commission's general directions into clear agreements among the affected parties with regard to implementation. It ruled that "the attack on the *Directions* on the ground of vagueness fails."

Finally, Doctors Hospital claimed that it had been treated unfairly because the commission had not made clear the case the hospital had to meet and the specific information it was expected to provide; the HSRC had not held hearings or given Doctors the opportunities it had given other hospitals to make its case. Following a lengthy review of the commission's procedures leading up to its *Notices* and *Directions* and the opportunities for input it had afforded Doctors Hospital, the court concluded that the commission "was obliged to give the applicant a fair opportunity to make its views known...before it issued the Directions, and it did so." The application was dismissed.

Wellesley Central Hospital, joined by three individual applicants, sought to quash the *Directions* applying to it on the grounds that the HSRC had exceeded its jurisdiction, was biased, considered extraneous and irrelevant matters in coming to its decisions, violated procedural fairness and fettered its discretion, and that the *Directions* were void due to uncertainty. The three individual applicants, gay persons infected with HIV then receiving services at Wellesley Central Hospital, claimed infringement of their religious freedom under the Charter of Rights and Freedoms through the transfer of relevant clinical programs from a secular hospital to a Roman Catholic one.

Addressing first the issue of jurisdiction — whether the commission had the power to compel a corporation that operates a public hospital to divest itself of its assets or to otherwise interfere with its property rights — the court pointed out, citing the ruling of Mr. Justice Campbell in the Pembroke case, that its only role was to decide if the HSRC had acted according to law in arriving at its decisions. After noting that "an urgent need to restructure and rationalize health services in Metro Toronto has been recognized for over a decade," the court reviewed the work of the Metro Toronto DHC, the legislative and regulatory powers of the commission, and the processes used by the commission prior to issuing its *Notices* and *Directions* affecting Wellesley Central. In deciding that the HSRC had acted within its powers in ordering the hospital to relinquish its programs, services and temporary use of its buildings to St. Michael's, the court relied heavily on its decision in the Doctors Hospital case: that ordering the temporary use of one hospital's buildings and assets by another was within the commission's powers. It also held that the order to negotiate an agreement with St. Michael's and the recommended disposal of the hospital's land, buildings and assets did not constitute expropriation of Wellesley Central's property.

In dealing with the allegation that the commission's *Directions* were void due to uncertainty, the court also relied on the Doctors Hospital decision and pointed out that hospitals are regularly engaged in restructuring and are experienced in doing the very things the HSRC was ordering them to do. Furthermore, the commission had issued guidelines, appointed a facilitator and demonstrated (as in Sudbury) that it was prepared to amend its *Directions* to accommodate alternative solutions developed locally. Viewed from the perspective of "a well-intentioned hospital," the *Directions* were not void due to uncertainty.

The third issue was that the commission had given excessive weight to the interests of Roman Catholic providers of health care. Here again, the court relied on the Pembroke decision: "The commission was entitled and required in the discharge of its duty to consider the appropriate role in local health care systems of denominational health care providers and it did not exceed its jurisdiction by doing so." The court rejected Wellesley Central's argument that the directions be quashed on the ground that the HSRC took into account extraneous (religious) considerations.

Charging procedural unfairness, Wellesley Central argued that the HSRC was quasi-judicial in nature and therefore bound by the rules of natural justice in its dealings with hospitals. The court found, however, as in Pembroke and with Doctors Hospital, that the commission was not a judicial or quasi-judicial body; it was a policy-making body charged with conducting a comprehensive review of the health care system in Ontario and with formulating guidelines and policies for implementing its policy decisions. Wellesley Central was entitled to, and received during 1996 and early 1997, a reasonable opportunity to submit extensive documentation and to state its case. No breach of procedural fairness was found.

Although the hospital did not allege actual bias, it argued that the relationship of five people to the commission's decisions constituted a reasonable apprehension of bias. One commissioner (Hart MacDougall) had chaired St. Michael's Hospital Foundation; another commissioner (Harry Jansson) had been on the board of a hospital that could be perceived as benefiting from the HSRC's decisions; a special adviser to the commission was associated with the latter hospital; a third commissioner (Dan Ross) was a member of a law firm that had once acted for St. Michael's; and the commission's chief executive officer had been president and chief executive officer of yet another hospital in Toronto. The court pointed out that MacDougall and Jansson had resigned from their positions before joining the HSRC and subsequently adhered to its conflict-of-interest guidelines; that neither the commission's chief executive officer nor the special adviser had a decision-making role; and that Ross practised in London, with a "Chinese wall" between his HSRC responsibilities and all hospital-related work by other members of his firm. It concluded that the lack of evidence of a closed mind rendered without merit the bias ground of the hospital's application.

The hospital also argued that the commission's decisions were invalid because it had failed to exercise independent judgment and shown itself willing to be dictated to by the Ministry of Health in giving priority to restructuring urban hospitals over rural ones. The court quoted testimony by the HSRC's chief executive officer that the commission had chosen to defer its decision bearing on a rural hospital in Lambton County so that it could consider the implications of the government's rural health policy then under development by the ministry. The court observed again that the need to rationalize health services in Metro

Toronto had been recognized as urgent for over a decade and the HSRC had responded appropriately. Therefore the assertion that the commission lost jurisdiction on this ground was also dismissed.

Finally, Wellesley Central Hospital and the three individual applicants, one an atheist, demanded that the HSRC's *Directions* be quashed on the ground that transferring programs, including the HIV/AIDS treatment programs, to St. Michael's would compel patients to seek health care in a religious environment at odds with their lifestyles, beliefs, sexual orientations and religions, and deprive women of abortions and related services. The court rejected the submissions on several bases. HIV/AIDS treatment programs and abortions were available in at least three other hospitals in the vicinity; no patient would be compelled to attend St. Michael's. In any event, as in Pembroke, "The silent presence of crucifixes does not constrain the chosen religious practice of those exposed to them and does not compel or coerce them to engage in religious practices or observances which they would not freely choose." The court also noted that the alleged breaches of patients' Charter rights had not occurred; they were prospective. This ground to quash the commission's *Directions* was also dismissed.

The failure of all of these applications to the courts seeking to quash the commission's *Directions* must have given pause to hospitals considering the same course of action. Although notice was given in October 1997 that Ottawa's Montfort Hospital had engaged legal counsel to consider a Charter challenge should the issues affecting it not be satisfactorily resolved, no court challenges were mounted for nearly a year.

HOTEL DIEU, KINGSTON

In September 1998 the court heard an application by the Religious Hospitallers of St. Joseph of the Hotel Dieu in Kingston to quash *Directions*, issued in July, ordering the hospital to collaborate with the Kingston General and Queen's University to develop a plan whereby it would relinquish its programs to the General and close as a public hospital by the end of October.[15] Much as in the agreement reached locally in Sudbury, the Hotel Dieu was to be given an opportunity to manage services remaining at that site, with compensation for its use, and thereafter manage an ambulatory-care centre to be established on a new site by May 2000. As in the arrangement that the commission had ordered for Wellesley Central and St. Michael's, the Hotel Dieu was to nominate a third of the members of the General's board.

The *Directions* were challenged on three grounds: that they were patently unreasonable in the absence of evidence that the commission's restructuring plan was viable; that they violated the Sisters' religious rights under the Charter of Rights and Freedoms; and that the HSRC had failed to consider provincial land use and municipal bylaws under the *Planning Act*.

In addressing the argument that the HSRC had to consider any and all difficulties that might be encountered in implementing its directions, the court referred to the Wellesley Central case: "Here, the Commission's Directions are not an end point in the restructuring process. They are but one step along the way. One must look at the Directions from the perspective of a well-intentioned hospital." It held that the *Directions* were not unreasonable considering the breadth of the commission's powers, that a change in the site of the new ambulatory-care centre could be accommodated and that the HSRC could amend or revoke its *Directions* if necessary.

The court also held that the *Directions* did not breach the Sisters' freedom of religion. They required only that Hotel Dieu cease to operate as a public hospital; the Sisters could continue to "minister to the sick poor who live in the north end of Kingston" using their assets and facilities in any way they saw fit except as a publicly funded hospital. And it found that the HSRC, while not obligated to do so, had considered matters related to provincial land-use policy and the *Planning Act* raised by the Hotel Dieu in a submission following the release, the previous February, of the *Notices of Intention to Issue Directions*. The application was dismissed.

The Religious Hospitallers of St. Joseph sought and were granted leave to appeal this decision to the Court of Appeal. They put forward four grounds of appeal: that the court had erred in failing to find that the commission was subject to the *Planning Act*; that its review of planning matters fell below the standard required by that Act; that it was patently unreasonable to expect them to "destroy" their hospital before it was known whether the restructuring plan could ever be implemented; and that the *Directions* interfered with their Charter rights.

The Court of Appeal unanimously dismissed the appeal.[16] Dealing with grounds one and two together, it ruled that the HSRC had exercised no authority related to the *Planning Act* — land-use planning — and that it neither was obliged to nor should have attempted to resolve problems that implementation of its *Directions* could cause with respect to this Act or any municipal zoning bylaw. It also rejected the unreasonableness ground: "To suggest that the directions are patently absurd because every conceivable contingency has not been considered and provided for is itself absurd. No project could proceed if it was a requirement of its implementation that it must proceed without variation or adjustment."

Nor did the Court of Appeal accept the claim that the *Directions* had the effect of turning the Hotel Dieu into a secular hospital, which would have violated the *Charter of Rights and Freedoms* and its guarantee of religious freedom. The court pointed out that the real effect of the HSRC's decision was that public funding of the hospital would be terminated. The Sisters' argument that public funding would have to continue because of the hospital's religious foundation "simply cannot withstand scrutiny."

The Sisters sought leave to appeal from the Court of Appeal's decision to the Supreme Court of Canada. The Supreme Court dismissed the application.[17]

DOUGLAS MEMORIAL, FORT ERIE

On another front, in November 1999 an application was brought before the Ontario Superior Court of Justice by Douglas Memorial Hospital in Fort Erie for an order to quash HSRC *Directions* imposing a governance structure on the hospital, making it part of the Niagara Health Care System.[18] Douglas Memorial objected to losing its autonomy as a rural hospital by amalgamating with St. Catharines General Hospital, Greater Niagara General Hospital, Welland County General Hospital, Port Colborne General Hospital, Niagara-on-the-Lake Hospital, Shaver Hospital and the Niagara Rehabilitation Centre. It argued that the Ministry of Health's *Planning Guidelines: Planning to Implement the Rural and Northern Health Care Framework* precluded the commission's directing it to amalgamate and to operate under a new corporate structure with a single vision, mission and set of core values; in addition, Douglas Memorial and two other hospitals would have to create standing committees of the new board to develop criteria for decisions on the elimination of in-patient or emergency services at any of the three sites[19] "which approval shall not be unreasonably withheld." Douglas Memorial claimed that the commission had discriminated against it by not following, in its review of the Niagara region, the processes specified in the planning guidelines for rural and northern hospitals and therefore had exceeded its powers.

Mr. Justice Hambly noted that the Rural and Northern Health Care Framework had been developed by the ministry at the request of the HSRC, did not constrain the commission from imposing new governance structures on hospitals and, furthermore, as an expression of ministerial policy, "strongly encouraged" common governance. The planning guidelines called for a two-stage process: identification of networks of rural and northern hospitals, and determination of the role to be played by each. Douglas Memorial claimed it was discriminated against because the commission had proceeded to include it in hospital restructuring for the whole of the Niagara Regional Municipality without first identifying it as part of a network. Mr. Justice Hambly ruled that the HSRC had not been discriminatory in terms of the process it used, had acted in good faith and in the public interest and had not exceeded its powers. The application was dismissed.

MONTFORT, OTTAWA

The last challenge to the commission's *Directions*, the only successful one and by far the most contentious and far-reaching in its implications, came out of hospital restructuring in Ottawa-Carleton, Canada's capital region. Its focus was the Montfort Hospital, a mid-sized community hospital that operated predominantly in French, providing primary and some secondary care mainly to the large francophone population of the city and townships extending east to the Quebec border.

Following its own review and that of the Champlain (Ottawa-Carleton) DHC of how and where hospital services were provided in Ottawa-Carleton, the commission issued its initial *Notices of the Intention to Issue Directions* in February 1997, nearly a year into its mandate. In this instance the DHC's report had not been very helpful. Despite a voluminous account of its data analysis and extensive consultations within the community, it fell short of recommending rationalizing the provision of services by Ottawa-Carleton's eight public hospitals: five acute-care (including a highly specialized pediatric hospital); one psychiatric/rehabilitation; and two complex continuing care facilities offering chronic care and long-term rehabilitation, palliative care and respite care. Basically, the DHC recommended maintenance of the status quo. In its *Notices* the commission signalled its support for consolidating the community's hospital services in five organizations: a single community/tertiary-care hospital arising out of the merger of three of the more specialized hospitals,[20] an acute-care community hospital in the city's rapidly growing west end, the pediatric hospital, a long-term mental health centre and a complex continuing care/rehabilitation centre.[21] Three of Ottawa-Carleton's smaller community hospitals,[22] including the Montfort, would be closed.

The commission's *Notices* provoked a storm of protest, not least from the francophone community, the DHC, the university and the Montfort itself. All urged the HSRC to preserve the only community hospital in Ontario operating in French, serving the large francophone population of the region and providing for the education of health professionals intending to practise in French. In coming to its final decision, the HSRC considered the many submissions it received on this subject with respect to Ontario's *French Language Services Act*,[23] which provides for the "designation" of hospitals (and other agencies) if their services are reliably available in French on a permanent basis. In Ontario there are no French or English hospitals; either hospitals are "designated" or they are not. In August the commission reversed its original intentions and ordered the Montfort to remain open, but primarily as an ambulatory-care hospital with a reduced number of beds (66), including 15 low-risk obstetrical beds, sufficient to accommodate a small number of deliveries, and 51 mental health beds. It also ordered the Montfort to take the lead in establishing a French Language Services Health Network in Ottawa-Carleton. And it ordered the amalgamated community/tertiary-care hospital, the Children's Hospital of Eastern Ontario and the Sisters of Charity facility to become fully "designated" hospitals under the Act — that is, capable of providing all their services equally in French and English.

As its *Notices* had done previously, the commission's *Directions* provoked a storm of protest, this time because of the perceived "downgrading" of the Montfort to an ambulatory-care hospital. Clearly, the HSRC's intention of having the Montfort play a leading role in defining the status of hospitals of the future, of changing the image of facilities with lots of beds from "kings of the hill" to "where the failures of ambulatory care go," was not appreciated. Over the next several weeks the commission amended its *Directions* to add 22 subacute beds, for a total of 88, at the Montfort, down from its original complement of 196.

But this was not enough. The hospital and several individuals applied to the court to have the commission's *Directions* set aside.[24] The hearing was originally scheduled for January 1999 but was postponed twice, first to permit the commission to consider advice from its Restructuring Coordinating Task Force in Ottawa and from educational consultants, who recommended the location of between 40 and 50 acute-care beds at the Montfort to support its academic mission. At around this time, the commission finally received confirmation of the ministry's rejection of its recommendation for a separate category of subacute beds — a decision that affected the Montfort. And finally, in May, the government removed the commission's power to issue *Directions,* leaving it, from that point on, capable only of recommending to the minister amendments to *Directions* issued previously.

In court, the Montfort Hospital and its co-applicants attacked the commission's *Directions* on three grounds. First they argued that they violated the equality rights of francophones under the Charter of Rights and Freedoms. The court rejected this argument on the basis that the equality-rights section of the Charter could not be used as a "back door" to enhance language rights beyond those specifically provided for elsewhere in the Charter. Then they argued that the *Directions* were patently unreasonable and therefore invalid. The court also rejected this claim, basing its decision on the previous judicial-review decisions recognizing the breadth of the commission's discretion and powers.

The third and most significant claim was that the *Directions* violated one of the *unwritten* structural or organizing principles of the Constitution, that of respect for and protection of minorities, in this case the francophone minority in eastern Ontario, representative of one of the country's founding cultures. The court accepted this submission and found that the Montfort's designation under Ontario's *French Language Services Act* gave the francophone community the right to receive health services in a "truly francophone environment," a right that included the facilities necessary for health care education and training in French:

> Directions which replace a wide variety of truly francophone medical services and training at Montfort with services and training elsewhere in a bilingual setting — however well those bilingual facilities may appear to work in any given case — fail to conform to the principle underlying our Constitution which calls for the protection of francophone minority rights. This is the flaw in the Commission's deliberations and in the directions emanating from them.

Accordingly the court quashed the *Directions* applying to the Montfort Hospital. This decision was subsequently appealed by the Province of Ontario, the commission by then having passed its sunset. The appeal was denied.[25]

OUT-OF-COURT SETTLEMENTS

A small number of other decisions came close to being challenged in court. Undoubtedly the nearest of these "near things" was the order for Toronto's downtown Women's College Hospital and Orthopaedic and Arthritic Hospital to merge with the Sunnybrook Health Sciences Centre, located in a more residential, northern part of the city, to form what has since developed into Sunnybrook and Women's Health Sciences Centre. It would be a gross understatement to say that neither of the two hospitals was keen to do so, but the more resistant by far was Women's College. Led by its politically connected and very determined chair, Jane Pepino, a lawyer, Women's College, joined by the O and A, did apply to the court to nullify the *Directions*, an application that was formally opposed by Sunnybrook, standing with the commission. From the start of the commission's review of hospitals in Metropolitan Toronto, Women's College dispatched to the HSRC an unrelenting stream of data, proposals and counterproposals over a period of years; its representatives demanded frequent meetings with the chairman, chief executive officer and senior members of the Metropolitan Toronto restructuring team, and when in-person meetings could not be arranged telephone meetings were held. A very effective public relations campaign kept the issue alive in the media for months. At the last moment, in fact the night before the scheduled start of court proceedings, an agreement was finally struck between Pepino and Mark Rochon, the commission committing itself to use its good offices to broker a mutually satisfactory deal among the parties and to issue a press release to that effect the following morning. The court was so advised, the press release was issued to a scrum on the courthouse steps, and an expensive and divisive court case was averted.

The commission devoted a great deal of time, effort and energy, as well as considerable sums of money, to the court challenges to its *Directions*. The fact that it withstood all but the last challenge to its authority and the processes and procedures it employed to reach its decisions is a credit to the commissioners and HSRC personnel; they took an open-minded approach to every option and problem and resolutely applied their three criteria — accessibility, quality and affordability — and their "man in the moon" test to every decision made. The advice of Hugh Kelly,[26] who was consulted as the commission began to develop its procedures, was good indeed; those procedures proved to be both sound and robust when examined in the courts. Greatly valued also were the wise counsel and inspired representation of John Laskin and his colleagues. Always readily available, they spent many hours educating the commission, particularly its chief executive officer and senior personnel, in the principles and requirements of administrative law as it applied to the HSRC's processes of consultation, deliberation and decision-making. Laskin's confidence was as vital as his knowledge and experience in supporting the commission through the unfamiliar processes of "discovery," factum writing and the like. His reputation as an extraordinarily successful litigator was an added advantage. Some individuals later confided that their institutions had decided not to challenge the commission's *Directions* in court because they did not want to "take on" John Laskin. The HSRC's "busy legal practice" could not have been better served.

NOTES

1 Laurentian Hospital and Sudbury Memorial Hospital.
2 Sudbury Algoma Hospital/Network North.
3 A former Ontario deputy minister of health.
4 "Canon law is the body of laws and regulations made by or adopted by ecclesiastical authority, for the government of the Christian organization and its members. The word *adopted* is here used to point out the fact that there are certain elements in canon law borrowed by the Church from civil law or from the writings of private individuals, who as such had no authority in ecclesiastical society. Canon is derived from the Greek *kanon* i.e. a rule or practical direction (not to speak of the other meanings of the word, such as list or catalogue), a term which soon acquired an exclusively ecclesiastical signification. In the fourth century it was applied to the ordinances of the councils, and thus contrasted with the Greek word *nomoi*, the ordinances of the civil authorities; the compound word 'Nomocanon' was given to those collections of regulations in which the laws formulated by the two authorities on ecclesiastical matters were to be found side by side" (Knight 2003).
5 *Connelly v. Ontario (Health Services Restructuring Commission)* [1997] O.J. No. 129 (Ontario Court of Justice [General Division], Divisional Court, Steele J).
6 *Ontario Public Services Employees Union v. Ontario (Health Services Restructuring Commission)* [1997] O.J. No. 2144 (Ontario Court of Justice [General Divison], Divisional Court, O'Leary J).
7 The submission also related to the Psychiatric Public Hospitals in London and St. Thomas.
8 *Pembroke Civic Hospital v. Ontario (Health Services Restructuring Commission)* [1997] O.J. No. 2749 (Ontario Court of Justice [General Division], Divisional Court, MacPherson J).
9 *Pembroke Civic Hospital v. Ontario (Health Services Restructuring Commission)* [1997] 36 O.R. (3d) 41 (Ontario Court [General Division], Divisional Court, Campbell, and Then and Matlow JJ).
10 *Pembroke Civic Hospital v. Ontario (Health Services Restructuring Commission)* [1997] 102 O.A.C. 207 (Ontario Court of Appeal, Goudge JA).
11 *Pembroke Civic Hospital v. Ontario (Health Services Restructuring Commission)* [1997] O.J. No. 3603 (Ontario Court of Appeal, McMurtry CJO and Robins and McKinlay JJA).
12 *Wellesley Central Hospital v. Ontario (Health Services Restructuring Commission)* [1997] O.J. No. 2752 (Ontario Court of Justice [General Division], Divisional Court, Hartt, McRae and Matlow JJ).
13 *Wellesley Central Hospital v. Ontario (Health Services Restructuring Commission)* [1997] 151 D.L.R. (4th) 706 (Ontario Court of Justice [General Division], Divisional Court, Southey, Boland and O'Connor JJ).
14 *Doctors Hospital v. Ontario (Health Services Restructuring Commission)* [1997] 103 O.A.C. 183 (Ontario Court of Justice [General Division], Divisional Court, Southey, Boland and O'Connor JJ).
15 *Russell v. Ontario (Health Services Restructuring Commission)* [1998] 114 C.A.C. 280 (Ontario Court of Justice [General Division], Divisional Court, MacFarland, Salhany and Sedgwick JJ).
16 *Hôtel Dieu Hospital of Kingston v. Ontario (Health Services Restructuring Commission)* [1999] 175 D.L.R. (4th) 185 (Ontario Court of Appeal, Finlayson and Weiler JJA and MacPherson J [ad hoc]).
17 [1999] S.C.C.A. No. 395.
18 *Douglas Memorial Hospital v. Ontario (Health Services Restructuring Commission)* [1999] O.J. No. 4516 [Ontario Superior Court of Justice, Hambly J]).
19 Douglas Memorial (Fort Erie), Port Colborne and Niagara-on-the-Lake.

20 The Ottawa General Hospital, the Civic Hospital and the Ottawa Heart Institute.
21 Respectively, the Queensway-Carleton Hospital, the Children's Hospital of Eastern Ontario, the Royal Ottawa Hospital and the Sisters of Charity of Ottawa.
22 The Riverside, Salvation Army Grace and Montfort Hospitals.
23 R.S.O. 1990, chapter F.32, guarantees each individual the right to receive provincial government services in French in 23 designated areas of the province.
24 *Lalonde v. Ontario (Commission de restructuration des services de santé)* [1999] 48 O.R. (3d) 50 (Ontario Court of Justice [General Division], Divisional Court, Carnwath RSJ and Blair and Charbonneau JJ).
25 *Lalonde v. Ontario (Commission de restructuration des services de santé)* [2001] 56 O.R. (3d) 505 (Ontario Court of Appeal, Weiler and Sharpe JJA and Rivard J [ad hoc]).
26 Of Miller Thompson, LLP.

CHAPTER 9

WHAT HAPPENED, WHAT DIDN'T, WHAT'S NEXT

As the commission pointed out in one of its last reports, "Improving performance requires action. It means going beyond what is wrong to actually doing things better and continually improving situations, relationships, programs and services. [It] incorporates the notion of accountability" (HSRC 2000d, 22). What about the commission's accountability? Did the HSRC's work lead to improved health care?

The HSRC was set up to restructure Ontario's public hospitals, to recommend strategies on how best to restructure other components of health care and to foster the creation of a genuinely integrated health-services system. Its principal purpose was to improve the functioning of hospitals and other health care contributors both individually and together.

Of the commission's achievements since March 1996, perhaps the most important is that, for a time at least, it broke the mould of the status quo ante. By exercising its power, the HSRC demonstrated that it *is* possible to make changes in health care — or at least to restructure hospitals. A goodly number of Ontario's urban acute-care hospitals have closed or are in the process of being closed.[1] A number of others have been joined together to form larger organizations that now provide services of higher quality, all without sacrificing their accessibility to the people and populations who need them. Most amalgamations and program transfers have unfolded as ordered by the HSRC. In some restructured hospitals, however, where receptivity to the commission's directions was low from the outset, the "friction cost" associated with making change has been high; Toronto's Sunnybrook and Women's Health Sciences Centre is one example. But, according to most reports, the majority of the institutions and communities affected by the commission's decisions consider themselves better off; they are not looking back yearningly to their past.

There are a number of outstanding success stories. In downtown Toronto the Centre for Addictions and Mental Health, created through the amalgamation of the Queen Street Mental Health Centre (a Provincial Psychiatric Hospital [PPH], the Donwood Institute, the Addiction Research Foundation Clinical Institute, the Mental Health and Addiction Services Corporation and the Clarke Institute of Psychiatry, is demonstrating effective leadership in bringing together all aspects of its coordinated mission. St. Michael's Hospital's integration of the programs offered to and populations served by Wellesley Central shows that the "takeover" of one hospital by another can sometimes be more effective than amalgamation. The University Health Network's incorporation into its Western Division the distinctive community-focused programs it inherited from Doctors Hospital demonstrates that an old organization can indeed learn new tricks. The HSRC's closure of some downtown Toronto hospitals is seen by most as a good thing; the shift of their capacity to other organizations and expansion of the scope of such services as cardiac care and cancer care has made those services more readily available in the city's periphery, where more and more people live.

Stronger, more robust community hospitals is a "big win" emerging from the restructuring process. Some District Health Councils (DHCs) have contended that a number of community hospitals would not have been able to survive the funding cuts of the late 1990s without joining forces with others. The several bigger, stronger community hospitals, offering increasingly sophisticated services, that were created by the HSRC in the "905" region — including Trillium Ridge, Sir William Osler, Markham-Stouffville and Lakeridge — although struggling to meet the needs of rapidly expanding catchments (as they will be for many years to come), are clearly on their way to high status among community hospitals. Windsor, Belleville, Milton, Oakville and many other communities are home to similar success stories. In Chatham, a Catholic and a secular hospital share a single building, showing that the new, integrated community hospitals can preserve the diversity of the founding institutions. This new breed of community hospital is taking on responsibility for the provision of more and more complex, sophisticated services previously available only centrally in the tertiary/quaternary hospitals of health-sciences centres. The competitive tensions for the recruitment of subspecialists and highly skilled nurses and other professionals arising from this shift flow from progress, as yesterday's tertiary services become secondary ones, moving out to where people live from the teaching hospitals, in which new, even more sophisticated (quaternary) services are being developed.

Ottawa's spectrum of restructured hospitals bears special mention, given the difficulties that the community, the DHC, the hospitals and the commission faced from the very outset until long after the *Directions* had been issued. The creation of a genuinely coordinated hospital system, increasingly linked — through the Community Care Access Centre (CCAC) — with home and long-term care, has taken longer than expected in Ottawa. Yet the way in which its eventual success has played out there sets an example for other communities.

In general, the two greatest barriers to operational/organizational change are the delay caused by insufficient capital and capacity constraints, particularly with regard to acute in-patient care. In communities where capital-construction projects have been completed, the program realignments/transfers ordered by the HSRC have also been completed. However, progress in implementing program realignments has been compromised in several communities as a consequence of delayed government decision-making with regard to the capital and operating funds necessary for restructuring. As for capacity, long delays in hospital admission remain a serious problem in many communities. As we have seen, the in-patient capacity constraints on acute care relate in large part to the shortfall of over 1,700 beds in the system — nearly 20 percent fewer than the HSRC's targets for 2003. This shortfall is a result of those hospitals having insufficient funds out of the hospital funding envelope to hire the nurses, aides, cleaners and other staff necessary to open the number of beds projected in the late 1990s by the HSRC to meet 2003 needs. It also appears, from the shrinkage in the number of acute-care beds between 2001 and 2003, that the pattern of hospital downsizing that preceded the commission's creation has continued past its sunset, and likely for the same reason — increases in the rate of demand for hospital-based services and hospitals' associated expenditures, notably increased wages and salaries, which have exceeded the rate of increase in their funding. It is not a healthy situation.

The capacity problem is compounded by the continued occupation of almost an equivalent number (1,565 as of March 31, 2003) of the existing acute-care beds by alternative level of care (ALC) patients. First, the commission's recommendation to the ministry that subacute beds be differentiated from acute-care beds was rejected; their quite different functions remain muddled. Second, although progress has been made in most communities, the government's commitment to the capital construction of new nursing-home, home-for-the-aged and continuing-care beds for ALC patients, expected to be in place by 2003, has been slow to come on line. While this expansion of residential capacity will certainly be needed as the population ages, the commission's advice to the government in 1998 was to give priority in the short term to less expensive (but also less politically visible) and more readily available "places" over "spaces," concentrating first on expanding services provided through home care, supportive housing and the like.

In communities where restructuring progress has been slower than anticipated or has been lacking, DHCs and others have cited a combination of factors:

> lack of government resolve combined with political interference
> lack of government leadership
> resistance by vested interests in the community
> lack of funding
> fundamental resistance to change
> community rivalries
> personal rivalries among hospital leaders at both board and management levels
> continued questioning of the appropriateness of the commission's *Directions*, relating especially to the number of acute-care beds assigned

On the government side of the ledger, memories of the fate of Frank Miller have been, if not erased, superseded by the reality of the 1999 election: changes in health care, extending even to hospital mergers and closures, are not necessarily the political equivalent of "touching the third rail." The optimistic view is that the changed hospital landscape may well embolden some future government (and perhaps even forward-looking, public-spirited health care providers acting from the bottom up) to initiate many of the other changes necessary to speed progress toward the creation of a genuine health care system. Pessimists would have it, however, that as time passes and the work of the commission fades to memory, the old mould, cracked but not broken, will repair itself and the (non)system's focus will revert to the single, simplistic question of how much more money its hospitals, physicians, home-care agencies, long-term-care facilities, drug companies and other providers must have year by year to maintain satisfactory levels of service under the status quo. For all the rhetoric to the contrary, and all the evidence that the status quo is unaffordable and comes with hugely damaging opportunity costs measured in terms of the sacrifice of other, more powerful, determinants of health (Conference Board of Canada 2004), so far the pessimists appear to be right. If they are, Ontario's Health Services Restructuring Commission will go down in history as a brave experiment that failed to generate the momentum necessary to sustain health care reform much beyond Ontario's urban hospitals.

Returning to the vexed topic of capital, large construction projects have been undertaken successfully in some communities. The majority, however, even those that are now complete, have taken much longer and cost much more than expected. In virtually all communities the level of capital reinvestment proposed by hospitals and provided by governments and private benefactors has greatly surpassed that recommended by the HSRC; those cost increases have strained the limits of what can be raised locally through fundraising campaigns and other means.[2] It is impossible to develop an "apples by apples" comparison of the HSRC's reinvestment targets and what has actually taken place, because most capital redevelopment projects differ radically from those ordered and costed by the commission; for the most part they encompass a much wider scope of capital redevelopment and expansion. In some communities (e.g., Sudbury and Oshawa) restructuring projects were begun and then put on hold by the ministry for extended periods as a result of cost overruns. In several communities the construction delays have overtaken the HSRC's 2003 bed-planning targets, and in some they have prevented the ordered consolidation and/or realignment of programs (e.g., in Sudbury clinical programs are still delivered at three separate sites pending completion of a new tower on the Laurentian Hospital site). The delay in capital redevelopment has also contributed to capacity problems and growing public concern about waiting lists. In some communities, delays have contributed to problems in "right sizing" capital projects, especially in communities such as the "905s," where population growth is particularly rapid.

Cost overruns have been troublesome both centrally, for governments, and locally, especially when they exceed a community's ability to raise the funds necessary to meet the government-mandated "local share." The growing dependency of worthy causes on charitable giving has "tapped out" many local donors and foundations. The municipalities concerned, already heavily committed to maintenance and renewal of their infrastructure and to social-support responsibilities "downloaded" to them in the 1990s, are chary of loading yet more on the property-tax base to cover the cost of renewing hospitals; they see health care as a provincial responsibility. After more than a decade of constrained funding, the historically low position of working capital within hospitals is at rock bottom;

hospitals are experiencing increasing difficulty in securing debt financing with their poor cash flow and the uncertainty of future provincial funding. Federal investment in hospital capital/infrastructure projects is minimal and the lack of experience with public-private partnerships precludes their adoption holus-bolus.

A contributor to the deficiency in operating funding has been what some hospitals describe as a fundamental flaw in the methodology used by the commission to calculate the savings that hospitals could achieve by restructuring. The budgets used as a base for those calculations of savings were those of the hospitals concerned prior to application of the government's mandated average cuts in 1996-97 and 1997-98 of 5 and 6 percent respectively. The hospitals claimed that this resulted in an 11 percent (on average) overestimate by the HSRC of the potential savings from their being restructured, an estimate inflated by the fact that cost-of-living increases for hospitals were not funded for the whole period. It is true that, without subsequent adjustment for the specific decrease in funding applied to each hospital individually, this methodology would have inflated the estimated savings gained from restructuring; it would have supported the ministry's decision to allocate funding well short of meeting their costs, much less than necessary to open and staff additional beds. Hospitals claim that by the time the ministry applied the HSRC's estimates, the savings were already gone. When the HSRC applied its cost-saving methodology, however, it had only the pre-1995-96 budget/expenditure data at hand; accordingly it did recommend to the ministry that the anticipated savings be recalculated once the actual data for each hospital were collected for the financial years concerned. Whether those recalculations were done or not was never reported to the commission. If they were not, the source of the observed funding discrepancy is clear. Application of the commission's methodology without subsequent adjustment of each hospital's actual base funding would have reduced the hospitals' operating budgets much more than the commission had intended or than was justified by restructuring.

Another outstanding issue in most communities is the perceived slow pace of reinvestment in the community sector, in expanding the capacity of mental health care, supportive housing and other community-based services, and especially home care. From the hospital and community perspectives alike, the funding available is insufficient to support changing caseloads, including those associated with population growth. Community-based care remains poorly linked to the hospital sector, where the absence of funding is said also to impede the application of best practices and desirable changes for the providers of alternative health services in the community. Generally speaking, reinvestment, including that recommended by the HSRC, has not significantly altered the balance between hospital and community-based service expenditures. In fact, the budgets of most community-based services have been flatlined for several years, while hospital budgets have increased. The greatest potential for decreasing the overall cost of hospital care lies in the continued application of new technology and knowledge (including pharmaceutical care) to enable hospitals to diagnose and treat more and more people as outpatients and to use their in-patient beds exclusively for those who cannot be cared for elsewhere.

The trend toward outpatient care cannot be optimized without reinvestment in community-based care. Nor can it be optimized without widespread dissemination of knowledge — through, for example, the publication of up-to-date reports[3] of small area variations in the rates and results of day surgery and other procedures that draw attention to advances made by leaders in the field and provide incentives for others to emulate and even outdo them. A related issue that remains to be addressed is shortages of health human resources, especially of nurses; in some areas this has restricted implementation of programs ordered by the HSRC.

Delays in implementing changes to mental health services are a particular problem in several communities. Delays most frequently mentioned include those in:

> establishing new adolescent mental health beds
> the ministry's responding to reports/recommendations submitted by the Mental Health Implementation Task Forces[4]
> proceeding with the divestment of PPHs in some communities and getting the ministry to "let go" in others[5]

Integration of the system as a whole is still a significant shortcoming everywhere, in particular integration of the primary-care function as the main "enabler" of integration across the care continuum.

Of the commission's two powers — decision-making and recommending policies for system building — far more has come out of the former than the latter. When restructuring hospitals, the HSRC had the power of decision. When the government finally took action, in 1998, on its recommendations to reinvest in the expansion of home care and long-term care, community by community, the principal barrier fell and the decisions affecting hospitals — especially those relating to governance and organization — were acted on fairly rapidly. In fact tremendous progress has been made generally in implementing changes in hospital roles and governance structures throughout Ontario's major urban areas. All of the *Directions* related to governance changes have been completed, with the notable exception of Kingston.[6] In most communities there is strong congruence between the progress made toward integrating all hospital-based services and the vigorous response of hospital boards to the challenge of realigning governance structures as the foundation for restructuring their hospitals and linking them with other local health-service providers. The changes related to essential capital reconstruction projects have taken much longer; some are still ongoing in 2005 and a few are just not happening at all.

Turning to an evaluation of the commission's performance, this can be divided into two categories: what succeeded and what did not. The processes the HSRC developed to support the first headlong phase of hospital restructuring, dependence on the previous work of the DHCs and an active search for evidence from the community in the form of feedback on its *Notices* prior to issuing its *Directions,* was successful. The commission reduced the risk of making wrong-headed decisions by relying on advice from those affected on what was possible locally and what was not. The avoidance of one-size-fits-all solutions was successful, judging by the fact that the great majority of restructured organizations are functioning well with nothing but happy memories and good traditions inherited from their antecedents. This outcome was facilitated by the commission's success in enlisting the enthusiastic support of community leaders, especially hospital and DHC leaders.

The HSRC's resistance to political influence, lobbying, protests and all manner of attempts to persuade it to modify its decisions was at odds with the influence game played by hospitals and the government. For nearly four years, evidence, complemented by reasoned argument based on knowledge of local conditions, was everything and influence was out! The commission's arm's-length relationship with government, though a success in some respects (as in removing influence from the equation and allowing it to come to decisions quickly), was a failure in others. The commission would have benefited from more interaction with politicians representing constituencies in which hospitals were being restructured. The biggest and costliest failure, however, was the inability of the minister and the ministry (and to some extent the DHCs) to meet the challenge of change. In struggling to implement the commission's *Directions*, the ministry was curiously unwilling to turn for help to the DHCs with their greater experience of local issues. In fact the DHCs drifted even further "out of the loop" throughout, and particularly following, the commission's four years. Some, as in Sudbury, where the hospitals do not even submit their operating plans or any other information to the DHC, appeared to be essentially disenfranchised before the closure of DHCs in 2005 — a senseless waste of expertise and experience. In addition, the ministry was either unable or unwilling to sell the HSRC's recommendations and shepherd them through the government's labyrinthine paths from approval to action. And the processes at work in that labyrinth have changed not a whit! The government made no accommodation for the changes occurring in the field. The HSRC's sunset in March 2000 left a harmful power and decision-making vacuum.

In terms of outcomes, there is no question that the commission served as a catalyst for change in health care. In no time at all it transformed from glacial to lightning speed the pace at which Ontario's public hospitals decided to reorganize, create new boards with new members, govern and manage differently, form mergers, shift programs, or even close their buildings and go out of business. The HSRC's decision-making forced good decision-making elsewhere that would otherwise have taken place haphazardly, slowly and painfully under the unrelenting pressure of funding constraints that had constituted the government's method of forcing change. As a result, hospitals in Ontario have moved, in a short period, toward a situation of much greater interdependence both with one another and with CCACs and the providers of other health services to the populations they serve mutually — toward horizontal and vertical integration. In short, they now see themselves as participants in a developing health care system.

The commission was also successful in persuading the government to put money derived from its reduction of the hospital envelope into long-term care and home care. The total reinvestment of $2 billion was decided on arbitrarily and was slow in coming, but it has helped to shift the focus from hospital-based to community-based care. To give credit where credit is due, the shift to out-of-hospital care was one of the declared intentions of Premier Harris's "Common Sense Revolution." While it would have been preferable for the government to strike a different balance between long-term-care "beds" and "places," substantial reinvestments *were* made — and in capital construction in hospitals as well — funds that otherwise might have been eaten up in eliminating the provincial deficit or bailing out hospitals that ran up deficits, a disturbing and increasingly frequent practice despite loud rote declarations each year that it is for the "very last time."

In addition, the restructuring of urban hospitals throughout Ontario was accomplished with limited disruption of the work and lives of hospital employees and medical staffs.

Turning to the list of failures, neither the government generally nor the Ministry of Health were prepared to work in partnership with the commission on communications or human resources issues. Regardless of whether this reluctance on the part of government is attributable to a perceived threat to its independence, it would have been helpful had the government reinforced the HSRC's actions in these two areas. It would have been especially helpful had the government been willing to "talk up" the vision of a genuine health-services system, or at least support the commission's efforts to relay the core message that "this is all about improving the health-services system, not about saving money."

Another failure, cited repeatedly, was the lateness of the government's decisions to reinvest "savings" from hospitals in community-based care and to modernize hospitals through massive capital investment/redevelopment. Had these reinvestment decisions followed closely on the heels of the release of the HSRC's *Directions* and recommendations, a great deal of morale-sapping uncertainty could have been avoided. The delay came at the high cost of diminished confidence, on the part of those affected and to some extent the general public, in the purpose of the whole exercise as something other than cost-cutting. One of the subsequent criticisms of the commission concerned the handling of capital. Aside from the expected complaints that the HSRC's estimates of the capital requirements of restructuring were too low, the apparent disconnect between the commission's recommendations and the government's subsequent spending decisions reinforced suspicions in every affected community regarding the old adage "When they say it's not the money, it's the money!"

The commission has to accept full responsibility for its naïveté, its failure to consider the reality of the political calendar and the amount of work it could reasonably achieve in the time available. Although it took into account, and acknowledged publicly, the fact that its powers of decision would not last long, it remains that the political winds shifted before the restructuring fleet was completely around the headland and into harbour; the rural and northern hospital networks got left behind. Had the HSRC engaged more staff and issued more *Directions* applicable to more hospitals and communities — especially with regard to the formation of networks of rural and northern hospitals — before the government lost its nerve, Ontarians dependent on the hospital sector of the putative health-services system would have been better served. On the other hand, setting a faster pace could well have been counterproductive; as it was, the commission's capacity to manage change was stretched to the limit. And then there was the rate at which the system could absorb change; given its previous unchanging nature, that, too, may have been at or beyond the HSRC's limit.

Also, had the HSRC been able to proceed more synchronously with phases I and II, it is possible that resistance, within and outside government, would not have had time to build and that some of its system-building strategies, especially those directed to health information management and primary-care reform, would have been implemented.[7] This was the commission's single biggest failure: It failed to persuade the government to proceed past hospital restructuring, first to develop a comprehensive health information management system and then to make fundamental organizational changes, including those pertaining to the provision of primary care, to take Tommy Douglas's second step — "the big thing we haven't done yet." Until some future government summons up the courage to take that step, the system will remain more illusory than real — and unaccountable, unmanageable, inefficient and unaffordable.

That said, it is unfair to hold the commission responsible for failing to get the Harris government and its bureaucracy to take on the daunting task of organizing the delivery of health services. The HSRC did its part and its collective conscience is clear. Its vision, strategies and guidelines remain sound, well argued and supported by such evidence as exists as to their workability and affordability. Together, these form a good game plan. But the creation of a genuine health care system is an all-consuming game, one that can be initiated and played only by the federal, provincial and territorial governments, together with the many providers of health services, for the benefit of the Canadian populations in the audience.

The commission's policy decision not to use its power to replace some hospital boards was, in retrospect, a mistake. Some of these boards are still struggling to establish genuinely unified governance as a result of the HSRC's failure to admit defeat in its efforts to join them with other boards dominated by members opposed to the commission's plan. These new consolidated hospitals would have been far better served had the commission been less patient and less tolerant of some of their predecessors' obstructive shenanigans. The HSRC should have selectively ordered more takeovers and fewer mergers.

From a financial perspective as well, hospital restructuring would have proceeded more effectively and smoothly had the pressures on hospitals imposed by the government's previous decision to cut their budgets serially by 5, 6 and 7 percent been coordinated with restructuring. This lack of coordination led to, among other things, the problems associated with the commission's use of flawed methodology to estimate the financial savings derived from hospital restructuring.

At least from the perspective of the affected hospitals, the commission's approach to estimating the capital cost of the new construction associated with restructuring was ineffective. The hospitals all maintained that the real costs greatly exceeded the estimates — "You didn't give us enough beds or money" was the usual refrain. Yet, as one observer from a DHC noted confidentially, "[Capital] estimates were at an altitude not practical. This has caused huge disruption; capital became and continues to be a real source of problems." Whether the estimates were too high, too low or — from the perspective of the rare disinterested, objective observer — just right, there is no question that the capital required to build and maintain the infrastructure of a hospital subsystem to suit the needs of the population is an issue that remains to be addressed. That challenge was not within the commission's mandate. The HSRC confined itself to estimating the capital investments necessary only to implement its restructuring *Directions*.

To sum up, as with most endeavours, the results are mixed. On the whole, though, the commission succeeded in its mandate to restructure Ontario's public hospitals and to develop do-able strategies to move toward the goal of a genuinely integrated health-services system. If those strategies have not enabled Ontario to move even to a first down, the HSRC can hardly be blamed; neither the government nor the "providers/players" has fielded a team.

Did Ontarians get their money's worth? Over four years the HSRC spent some $16 million; about half of that amount went on staff salaries and benefits and on consulting, legal, financial and other services; the rest was spent on travel, general services, supplies and equipment, and the research for and preparation of the reports associated with phase II. The commissioners' honoraria came to a total of $41.[8] It is impossible to put a dollar value on the benefits of enhanced quality and affordability that will accrue over the long term from the restructuring of the province's urban hospitals and from the increased capacity of community-based long-term and home care. It is also impossible to estimate the benefits that could flow eventually from strategies to lay the ground for health information management, primary-care reform, performance evaluation, greater accountability and bottom-up integration — all those elements that are essential in transforming the field of silos into a true health-services system. The value of the real and potential benefits is substantial. It constitutes a significant rate of return on the investment of

$16 million to catalyze change in a (non)system that in 2002 consumed in excess of $43 billion in constant (inflation-adjusted) dollars, or $3,600 for each man, woman and child in Ontario (Statistics Canada/Canadian Institute for Health Information 2003). The commissioners can rest easy in the knowledge that they have given their all in fulfilling their mandate and delivering the best products they could given the constraints of time, paucity of data and lack of enthusiasm for change.

WHAT'S NEXT?

To quote Yogi Berra, "Making predictions is very difficult, especially about the future." But it is likely that most of the commission's *Directions* will stick. Over the long term, the newly created consolidated hospitals in urban centres will go from strength to strength. Their enhanced governance will grow stronger and become more representative of the populations they serve. They will build on their capacity for health information management and, led by a stronger, more active and more effective OHA, they will become more accountable and more "public" with the greater use, sophistication and comprehensiveness of "report cards," "performance agreements" and the like. The restructured hospitals will gradually generate performance data that will form the basis of a gold standard for reliably and cost-effectively meeting the needs of their populations for high-quality comprehensive services. Implementation is taking longer than expected, and undoubtedly the political will to be resolute in the face of continued opposition will wax and wane; if some changes to the commission's model are made, these will constitute but minor perturbations to the fundamentally restructured provincial hospital landscape. Among hospitals — and with respect to their relationships with providers of home care, long-term care and other services, including primary care — the shift from autonomy to interdependence will continue gradually but inexorably, driven by many factors, not least the demand by patients and their families for improvements in their continuity of care. The shift will be driven also by continued constraint in funding from the public purse, which will force hospitals and other providers to substitute lower-cost for higher-cost services whenever and wherever possible — and in ways previously thought impossible. It is also likely that hospitals and other publicly funded providers will face labour unrest as a result of the need to eliminate the now almost traditional differential between increases in rates of pay and increases in revenue growth.[9]

Elsewhere in the system, primary-care renewal will likely hobble along. The semi-independent shepherd of this work in Ontario, the Family Health Network — whose mandate was scheduled to end in March 2004 and was then extended to August 2004 — has been folded into the Ministry of Health after three years, having never really freed itself from its bureaucratic chains. And there are no signs that primary care will soon escape its doctor-centricity, growing inaccessibility, shrinking range of services, or increasing concentration in cities huddled beneath the skirts of specialists and hospitals dedicated to the care of the very ill and the injured. There are grounds for believing that health information systems will generate useful data that will, in fact, support continuity as responsibility for each patient's care shifts from one provider to another, as the patient goes from primary to acute care to rehabilitation to home care to long-term care. If the present overblown concerns about confidentiality can be overcome, the electronic patient record may well develop in the foreseeable future into a sharable tool to facilitate continuity of care; it may also become a means for the system and taxpayers to measure the real health benefits (as opposed to mere throughputs) of all that money spent on health services — all coupled with the capacity for increased rather than decreased personal privacy.

The improvements in health information management remain poorly coordinated — in fact, they are not really being managed at all — but they are taking place slowly and along similar lines throughout Canada, driven by three factors:

> the need for increased use of technology (software and hardware), given its availability and its performance in raising productivity in other fields
> the growing imperative of greater accountability and demonstration of money well spent
> the large sums being spent on "health infostructure" by the federal and provincial/territorial levels of government

What's next? What should we do to speed the conversion of the field of silos in Ontario into a real health-services system accountable to the people it serves? Had the HSRC been asked for its advice at its sunset in March 2000, it would have urged the following on government, health care providers, and the people who both benefit from and pay for health care:

> Apart from funds earmarked for "buying change" ("upfront" nonrecurrent expenditures), funding increases for health care should not exceed the rate of increase in the consumer price index or the gross domestic product or, perhaps, the government's tax revenues for the foreseeable

future. Funding increases over and above inflation, derived from any source, have been demonstrated in Canada and elsewhere to support the status quo and inhibit innovation and increased productivity.

> Government should get out of the management business. It should devolve *all* of its managerial authority and functions to such bodies as Regional Health Authorities (RHAs) or, better yet, Integrated Health Systems (IHSs), charged with funding and coordinating the delivery of *all* health care in their jurisdictions, including that provided by physicians and cancer and mental health services — all the sacred and secular cows in one herd. The other provinces and territories have a head start on such devolution, a process comprising three simultaneous steps: (1) as the capacity of RHAs and IHSs is built up, their managers gain experience and providers are weaned off direct interaction with the Ministry of Health; (2) sufficient capacity in health information management is achieved to support effective and efficient health care delivery within each RHA or IHS and the reporting relationship to the government to ensure accountability in terms of cost-effectiveness; and (3) the ministry is downsized and redesigned for its new role as support for the governance of the system.

> Government should concentrate on governing and on evaluating the performance of the evolving health care system. Its role should be to articulate its vision of the system and its values; establish the policy framework and guidelines necessary for RHAs and IHSs to manage health care delivery within their jurisdictions in order to fulfill that vision; provide envelope (as opposed to line-by-line, or earmarked) funding from the public purse; and evaluate and report to the legislature and the public on the progress being made.

> For the implementation of steps two and three, which should take between five and ten years, an interim successor to the HSRC should be established, funded by government but at arm's length from it, with responsibility for managing the transition and the evolving health-services system. Without such a body capable of insulating itself from the pressure tactics that so hobble political/governmental processes in contemporary society, true reform of our cherished health care system will take so long that before much progress has been made the political support of the middle class for its public funding may well be lost.

NOTES

1 As of March 2004 a total of 10 hospitals had been closed, although most had yet to be decommissioned.
2 Currently, the Ministry of Health expects that hospitals will contribute between 25 and 50 percent toward capital infrastructure and 100 percent toward the purchase of some medical equipment and ICT assets.
3 Such as those of the Institute for Clinical Evaluative Sciences.
4 Most communities that established Mental Health Implementation Task Forces have completed reports and submitted recommendations/plans to the ministry but are awaiting the ministry's approval and direction on how to proceed with mental health reform in their communities.
5 Despite official divestment, the ministry is still trying to exert some degree of control over services and beds (e.g., in London).
6 Where a single governance for acute-care services has not been established as directed by the HSRC for the Kingston General Hospital and the Hotel Dieu.
7 Ontario's Family Health Network initiative relates more directly to models developed jointly by the Ontario Medical Association and the Ministry of Health than to the HSRC's recommended strategy for reform of primary care.
8 Some were appointed for less than the full four years.
9 British Columbia in April/May 2004 provides a case in point.

CHAPTER 10

LESSONS LEARNED

Serving on the commission, whether as a commissioner or as a staff member, was a learning experience *sans pareil*. It was undoubtedly similar for the hospitals and communities affected by the commission's decisions, and perhaps also for the staff of the Ministry of Health and the government. Nothing like the HSRC had been done before and, as with all new things, it had many lessons to teach.

The lesson that took pride (or shame) of place at the top of the list, at least from the commission's perspective, was the difficulty of convincing vested interests, primarily health care bureaucrats and providers (including hospital governors, directors and trustees) that change should be considered not as a threat but as an opportunity to be seized and embraced as the way to a better and more secure future. History is replete with examples of once thriving enterprises, societies even, withering and dying after shifting their focus from a quest for improvement to mere preservation of the status quo. So it could be with our vaunted health care system in these early years of the twenty-first century. (Again, Dr. Arnold Aberman's quip comes to mind. Question: How many doctors does it take to change a light bulb? Answer: Change?) The commission concluded its legacy report, *Looking Back, Looking Forward,* with the slogan "Built to last means built to change" (Meyer and Davis 1998). Perhaps it should have used the more graphic maxim "If you're not prepared to drive the steamroller of change, get ready to become part of the road!"[1]

The commissioners were not naive. All had long experience in various fields of endeavour and were well acquainted with the strengths and foibles of human nature and organizations. But all were distressed at the depth and ferocity of the resistance to change among so many health care participants, not only providers but also the owners/governors and managers of health care's many institutions and organizations, including the government bureaucracy. It quickly became obvious that this aversion to change was graduated, its intensity being directly correlated to the objector's position on the funding ladder and his/her degree of autonomy, status and control vis-à-vis other health professionals, workers, organizations or institutions. These structures remain hierarchical, a feature of the "field of silos"; they constitute a compelling argument for a more equitable system respectful of the contributions of every silo, tall and short. Those standing on rungs nearest the top — mainly hospital boards and managers — thought of change as a losing proposition. Those lower down — home-care agencies, nursing homes and homes for the aged, for example — saw it as a good thing likely to help them ascend the ladder. What the commissioners found most irritating was the thin rhetorical cloak of altruism — "our concern is for the best interest of our patients" — glibly thrown over self-interested opposition to and support for change, whether by those speaking for institutions, health care professionals or employees seeking better working conditions. Patients and their families and the populations from which they are drawn seem far from the centre of our constellation of health services.

 Resistance to the changes ordered and recommended by the commission was far from universal. Many hospitals strongly supported the HSRC and its purposes, including hospital restructuring. The Ontario Hospital Association found itself unable to speak with one voice on the issue. While the Ontario Medical Association remained officially neutral, the Ontario College of Family Physicians expressed its strong support for the commission's strategy for the reform of primary health care, as did many individual physicians, especially those practising in small communities. That support, however, was attacked vigorously by the Coalition of Family Physicians, a large self-described splinter group pursuing its own agenda, comprising some general practitioners and family doctors practising in large cities, particularly Toronto. At the outset the Ontario Nursing Association, like unions representing hospital workers, suspected that restructuring would result in fewer jobs for its members, whereas the Registered Nurses Association of Ontario, with its somewhat different focus and interests, was more supportive — strongly so of the commission's strategy with regard to primary health care and its emphasis on greatly enhanced roles for nurse practitioners and nurses.

In 1998 William Thorsell, editor-in-chief of *The Globe and Mail*, wrote, "The phrase 'change for the better' is an oxymoron in the Canadian psyche" (Thorsell 1998). There were many times over their four-year mandate that the commissioners feared this to be true. But, in fact, to the extent it was able to gauge the reaction of men and women on the street to the changes it was ordering in hospitals and the recommendations it was making to the government, the commission was heartened. There was no widespread opposition to its *Notices* and *Directions*; in fact there were many spontaneous expressions of public support for its work. Although far from a referendum on hospital restructuring, the 1999 election appeared to confirm the point: the commission's decisions did not seem to have a negative effect on the government's prospects for re-election, even in ridings where the governing party feared the worst. It did not even appear to be an issue in the campaign; if it had, of course, the commissioners would simply have refused to be drawn into debate. The HSRC was encouraged to think that Thorsell, if not entirely wrong, was far too sweeping in his characterization of the public's attitude toward change, at least with respect to health care in Ontario.

Were the politicians too timid? Were they wrong to view health care change as equivalent to the proverbial third rail? Did they misread the public's perception of the need for hospital restructuring, primary-care reform, integration of health care silos, and the collection and management of health information in order to enhance governance, management and accountability? The election results suggest that the citizenry was quite prepared to endorse rather more dramatic and decisive actions than their political leaders were prepared even to contemplate. As it knew it would from the beginning, the Harris government wore the political consequences of the HSRC's every direction and recommendation. But at least the *Directions* wore well! The strategy of putting the commission at arm's length, insulated from the influence of politicians, was an effective one, for the HSRC could make decisions that the government itself could not, at least not in a timely fashion. But the HSRC could not distance the government from the possible political consequences. The commission took three lessons from the experience:

> Use of arm's-length bodies such as the HSRC is an effective way of making changes in public enterprises like health care, especially if those changes are urgently needed. It may not be the only way to make such changes, but, short of the kind of severe and prolonged crisis that forces political considerations into the shadows, it may be the timeliest and

most effective. Certainly that was the commission's conclusion when it recommended that the government appoint relatively independent bodies to implement its strategies for health information management and renewal of primary care.

> Delegating decision-making authority to such bodies does not diminish political accountability. Whether the delegate is a one-off organization like the HSRC, with a specific, circumscribed mandate, or a Regional Health Authority (RHA), Integrated Health System (IHS) or mental health agency — permanent organizations with managerial responsibilities — the government cannot, nor should it try to, divorce itself politically from the consequences of decisions made by its delegates.

> Governments' currently feeble approach to governance — leadership through policy direction and evaluation of outcomes — would be greatly enhanced by the use of arm's-length bodies, a genuine devolution of responsibility and authority to organizations more sharply focused on the issues at hand and, in the case of RHAs and IHSs, closer to the people affected by their decisions. Such devolution[2] would allow, even require, governments to concentrate more on governance/leadership — *what* is to be done and the *results* — and less on managerial issues — *how* it will be done, issues better handled by people on the ground. As it is now, governments and their bureaucrats are too far removed from the "workface" to manage properly the delivery of health services.

Another important tactical lesson was that it is vital to act quickly. Many considered the commission's pace from the beginning of phase I to be irresponsibly hectic. As it turned out, however, when the government took away the HSRC's power to order hospital restructuring, substantial work remained to be done, notably the creation of disciplined networks of small rural and northern hospitals. Despite the ministry's policy guidelines calling for the creation of such networks, without the force of direction very few were formed.[3] More seriously for the system, the commission's more policy-oriented strategies related to system building, health information management, transformation of primary-care delivery, and enhanced accountability through the measurement and evaluation of outcomes foundered on the shoals of political practicality. By the end of the HSRC's mandate the government's navigators were far more concerned with the issues themselves than with finding channels through or around them. Political history shows us that, except under the stimulus of a catastrophe like a war or the Great

Depression, rapid changes to the status quo can be made only by a newly elected government with a large majority; the newness to power ensures its idealism and zeal, while a healthy majority reinforces its courage. But 18 to 24 months in power may be the maximum — not nearly long enough to conceive and implement major changes to a system as large, complex and politically precious as health care. The HSRC could have engaged more commissioners and hired more staff and consultants, worked more quickly, and taken on phases I and II concurrently, but then the whole thing might have turned into *Mission Impossible*.

The downside of acting quickly, something the HSRC experienced as a result of its rapid pace, is that the system contains few people who know how to implement change of the kind and magnitude that it ordered and recommended. It is one thing to conceive of ways to improve things; it is quite another to make those improvements, especially when the majority do not entail capital investments in new construction or new equipment but require people to change their modus operandi. Changes of that nature — and most of those necessary to convert health care's silos into a system are of that nature — require a number of dedicated, experienced leaders willing to champion change. Although the commission did find champions in hospitals, on hospital boards, in District Health Councils (DHCs), and in the home-care and long-term-care sectors, their numbers were small. Also, the political, financial, cultural, religious and regulatory obstacles were too numerous and daunting to support rapid change solely from the bottom up. Decisive, forward-looking governance with a strong vision is essential to support those local champions of change and help them to enlist others in their ranks.

One of the obstacles to change is the regulatory environment — primarily the rules attached to government funding via the Ministry of Health. Meant to ensure that money is spent wisely, well and in strict accordance with the intentions of the legislature,[4] in many cases anticorruption safeguards, such as the parliamentary vote system, do not really foster accountability but have the effect of stifling local initiative and reducing local decision-makers to mere ciphers administering the straightjacket of line-by-line budgets or, at most, budget categories. Providing hospitals with global budgets coupled with alternative accountability mechanisms has been one attempt to foster both flexibility and local initiative. But global budgets have not extended far beyond hospitals, and even hospitals are not free of constraints when shifting their funds from one budget category to another; and hospitals, as their deficits illustrate, are restricted by policy in cutting service levels to fit the cloth of their funding.

While it is important to prevent fraudulent use of the public purse, governments' fear of criticism by their auditors general must not be allowed to obscure the goal of public spending: to achieve maximum benefit for the population under the circumstances that apply at the workface. The commission observed that too many of the rules and regulations defined by the centre were of the one-size-fits-all variety, so that responsible people on the ground were not given the latitude either to adapt to local circumstances in a timely fashion or exercise their ingenuity and provide innovative solutions to local, district or regional problems. Command-and-control management does not have a good track record, in health care or anywhere else.

The commission also learned, through the process of hospital restructuring, that large-scale change is possible — today's urban acute-care-hospital landscape in Ontario is quite different from that of 1996. Notwithstanding the lessons learned from this difficult experience, it demonstrates that fairly rapid change is possible in health care, given the political will and the right mechanisms. But changes of the nature tackled by the HSRC rest on a number of conditions.

CONDITIONS FOR CHANGE

The first condition is a powerful impetus for change. The HSRC served as the change agent for hospital restructuring, armed as it was, between 1996 and 1998, with the power of the government itself over hospitals, constrained only by the requirement that it act within the law and in the public interest. Those affected discovered quickly that the commission and its *Directions* were not subject to political influence or other kinds of pressure. Only one of the HSRC's decisions was successfully challenged in the courts. The commission was a highly visible and powerful force for change.

The second condition is that the purpose of change be clearly specified and be understood both by those directly affected and by the general public. While the commission's vision of a true health care system, with the population served at its centre, may well have been useful, the purpose of its hospital restructuring work was obvious from its mantra — quality, accessibility, affordability. Continued access to hospital-based services was very much on people's minds. For the public, as for the commission, proximity to a hospital was not much of an issue in cities, even in the Toronto megalopolis, where transportation services are readily available and relatively weatherproof. Several groups tried to make it an issue, but the commission's main concern in cities was to ensure that the fewer large hospitals whose creation it ordered have the capacity to provide timely, high-quality services to all who legitimately sought access to them. People also followed the logic of "those who do things frequently get better results than those who do them infrequently" — the commission's rationale for consolidating urban hospitals into a fewer, larger organizations in which the quality of care would be safeguarded and enhanced by virtue of scale. They also saw the wisdom of concentrating reinvestments in capital assets in such a way as to benefit from economy of scale. Although the criterion of affordability — "saving the government money" — would have been insufficiently compelling in itself to attract wide public support, it was compelling when linked with the other two criteria, quality and accessibility. People's tax bills are not irrelevant. Although it was not a major issue, the public viewed maintaining large numbers of empty beds and duplicating services in half-empty hospitals but a stone's throw apart as an inefficient way of providing valuable services that were threatened by their high costs. Articulation of the commission's purpose — *to maintain accessibility and enhance the quality and affordability of hospital-based services* — constituted a vitally important condition for change.

The third condition is persistence — staying focused on the goal and the long-term benefits of the change. Leadership of the Ministry of Health has been subject to repeated upheaval over the decades as ministers and deputy ministers (and other bureaucrats) have come and gone with distressing frequency, many arriving with very focused mandates they have been unable to fulfill before moving on. Ontario's hospitals have witnessed a succession of ephemeral fads (zero-based budgeting, management by objectives and the like) and have an understandably jaded response to new initiatives. The government's announcement of the HSRC's mandate and the legislated assurance that it would remain in place for four years notwithstanding any changes in the ministry created an important condition for change. This was reinforced by the commission's frequent restatement of its three criteria and its consistency in applying them to hospital restructuring, community by community, and later to its system-building policy work.

The fourth condition bears on the last point. The commission was handicapped in executing its mandate to restructure hospitals by virtue of the fact that a separate but highly relevant policy decision had been made prior to its creation — hospital budgets would be reduced by 18 percent (by 25 percent with inflation thrown in) between 1996-97 and 1998-89.[5] Although a funding-equity-based formula was used to avoid an indiscriminate across-the-board jolt to every hospital's financial status quo, it would have been far preferable had this fiscal policy been synchronized with the restructuring process itself; it should have been folded into the HSRC's criterion of affordability, permitting the exercise of greater discretion and selectivity in its application — a much more cleanly targeted approach. While a "burning platform" was necessary to stress the urgency of hospitals' making major changes, the government's prior announcement of its massive funding cut set everything ablaze, obscuring the commission's signposts that its *Directions* were the way to run. The slowness of the government's subsequent decisions on reinvestment in out-of-hospital services added fuel to the fire. It is important that everybody involved in ordering and implementing change be on the same page of the same songbook.

The fifth condition for successful change is the involvement of community leaders and, with respect to hospitals, local experts familiar with operational constraints and knowledgeable about what can and cannot be done. In this the commission was well served — even if somewhat variably — by the DHCs that had preceded it in their reviews of hospital-based services. Most had engaged community leaders, hospital and health care experts, and many citizens in public consultations on the development of options reflecting some hard decisions. The HSRC built on that work as it actively engaged people from the DHCs, the hospitals, other health care providers and their organizations, municipal and other elected officials, and media representatives in the development of its *Notices* and final *Directions*. Without the support of community people knowledgeable about local and other practical constraints but convinced of the necessity and wisdom of change and the benefits to be derived from the specific changes under consideration, little of consequence is likely to happen despite the power of central direction. Such people are scarce in hospitals and health care generally; in Ontario their enlistment is urgently required. The most effective approach to change is bidirectional — push and pull, bottom up and top down.

From its practice of appointing experienced outside facilitators (described in chapter 3), the commission learned the importance of making help available to local people in developing appropriate processes and negotiating change. The commission's facilitators demonstrated their critical role time and again, helping people to put long-standing differences behind them, to overcome all manner of obstacles and to progress toward agreement on implementing the changes ordered by the HSRC. Without the facilitators, decisions in many communities would never have been negotiated in a timely manner.

Finally, a vital condition for successful change is full awareness by those affected of what is intended and what is occurring. This condition can be met only through open, full, consistent and frequent communication. The commission learned that, however compelling the message from the perspective of the commissioners and staff, the work could not speak for itself. Its decisions, and the evidence and approaches that had led to them, had to be sold — in as many ways as possible. Early on it became apparent that despite meetings with editorial boards, media conferences, one-on-one media interviews, public announcements, and meetings with civic and political leaders, the commission's message either remained unclear or became garbled to the point of misinformation. Accordingly, the HSRC opted to purchase advertising space in local papers to ensure that everyone affected by its *Notices* and *Directions* had access to relevant and accurate information. It is wrong to impose change on the uninformed and the misinformed. All those affected must be informed of the purpose of the change, the means of change and the benefits to be expected from the change. It is difficult to reach all the diverse audiences in every community, but successful change demands that it be done.

LOCAL LEADERSHIP

Another lesson to be learned from the HSRC's experience is that deciding *what* to do is usually less difficult than deciding *how* to do it — in other words, easier said than done. As with the commission's *Directions*, the "saying" was done centrally (though every effort was made to accommodate particular community circumstances) and the "doing" locally. The HSRC considered it essential to enlist and retain the support of local hospital leaders, municipal officials and other prominent members of the community in order to have them champion the implementation of its *Directions*. It worked hard to maintain communication with the "doers" in every community in which it worked on hospital restructuring and to support them in every way possible. In this regard, the HSRC's facilitators were invaluable to both the commission and the community, especially in helping to develop communication and negotiation processes appropriate for the subculture of each community. Getting those processes right

— instilling confidence in the participants regarding their fairness and inclusiveness — was vital to compromise and the key to reaching agreement. There were times when the commission and its facilitators were frustrated to the point of exasperation that unresolved issues, even the time necessary to follow procedural steps in a drawn-out but agreed-upon process, got in the way of good decision-making. But in addition to the lesson that deciding how to make change is the hardest part of the process, it also learned that patience is a virtue and that perfecting the process leading up to change is absolutely essential.

The commission learned that there are striking differences in the cultural underpinnings of Ontario's many communities, regions and districts. These differences are apparent in large cities to be sure, but nowhere are they more so than in small communities, some of them not far distant from one another. Although demographically similar, a number of communities were the scene of heated public reaction to the idea of a hospital's even networking with one in a neighbouring town. The merger of hospitals in Port Hope and Cobourg is a case in point.[6] Whatever the perspective — civic pride, long standing rivalry, the recruitment of replacement physicians, the attraction of new businesses and industry — community culture means different things to different people. It is important to just about everybody and is not "manageable" in the sense of amenable to change, except perhaps by propinquity, mutually beneficial experience and "the tincture of time."[7]

Among expressions of religious diversity, the commission learned the significance of canon law (ecclesiastical law)[8] in dictating what could and could not be done with respect to partnering Roman Catholic hospitals with others and integrating them into a system of hospitals. The HSRC recognized from the outset the significant contributions of religious hospitals — Roman Catholic, Salvation Army, Jewish and Seventh Day Adventist — to the development of hospital care in Ontario and elsewhere. Many of the country's earliest hospitals were established by religious orders and operated by nursing sisters, and many of those orders continue to own the hospitals and to participate in their governance. The commission was never of the mind that homogeneity among hospitals is a good thing and was eager to preserve their diversity of cultures and traditions within an increasingly coordinated or integrated system of hospitals. It discovered early on that this ambition struck a chord with the majority of those in charge of hospitals; most were willing to find new, imaginative ways to integrate the work of their hospitals with that of others, but in ways that accommodated and preserved their distinctive religious cultures and values. This attitude of openness characterized the commission's discussions with representatives of all religions but these discussions quickly came up against the roadblock of canon law, which, according to its interpreters, expressly forbids the sharing of the governance or management of Roman Catholic and secular organizations. This was exemplified in a private conversation between the HSRC's chair and chief executive officer and a couple of Sisters representing an order. When asked what solutions might be available to resolve a particularly divisive issue, one of the Sisters said: "The Sisters…are not in the business of dividing communities! Leave this with us. We will find a solution. We ask only one thing — that you not tell 'the boys' what we're doing." "The boys" was a reference to the Church's male hierarchal interpreters of a canon law far less flexible than the great majority of those it binds. The governance options developed by the commission to overcome that inflexibility, Joint Executive Committees foremost among them, were never formally approved by Church authorities and have yet to stand the test of time. If they are not effective at what they are now being used for — to coordinate the activities of secular and religious hospitals — then the sacrifice over the long term may well be religious hospitals and hospital diversity itself.

The commission learned the futility of trying to forge workable, lasting partnerships among those fundamentally opposed even to their consideration. It went to great lengths, in several instances, to ensure the continued participation of two or more hospitals in joint endeavours, only to be frustrated by the obviously grudging nature of the collaboration that came out of prolonged, difficult negotiations extending to trivial points in the economists' category of "the least order of smalls." Given the opportunity to reconsider some hospital mergers, the HSRC would no doubt opt for takeovers and closures rather than try to unite unwilling partners.

QUANTITY/QUALITY

Finally, a bitter lesson for the commission was the degree to which the provision of highly sophisticated hospital services trumps the risk to patients of doing too few procedures, or seeing too few patients with similar problems to safeguard the quality of their outcome (the concept of critical mass). The point is illustrated by two cases that arose relatively late in the HSRC's mandate.

It was clear both from its own reviews and from the work of Ontario's highly respected and effective Cardiac Care Network that the provincial capacity for diagnostic and therapeutic angiography had to be expanded to accommodate the growing number of patients who could benefit from this expensive but effective procedure. An additional factor was that whereas angiography had been developed as a tool for determining the extent of occlusion of coronary (and other) vessels, interventional cardiologists were, increasingly, following on their diagnosis directly in the same procedure with arterial dilatation and stenting, an alternative to the riskier and even more expensive coronary artery bypass grafting. Given the issue of time-to-treatment, there was a good case for locating angiographic suites in every major population centre, a move advocated by even medium-sized hospitals eager to gain the prestige of possessing the capacity for such sophisticated work and thus attracting more doctors, particularly specialists. There were downsides, however, not least the limited supply of interventional cardiologists and the considerable expense of building, equipping and running the necessary facilities. But the key limiting factors were two: the availability in the same hospital of the facilities and personnel required for open-heart surgery in the event of accident or failure of therapeutic angiography, and calculation of the volume of cases necessary to ensure safety and high quality of outcomes under the "those who do them frequently do them better" principle.

After a thorough examination of all the issues and discussions with representatives of the Cardiac Care Network, the commission came to the conclusion, based primarily on safety considerations, that the expansion of cardiac angiography to include therapeutic interventions (dilatation and stenting) should be confined to those hospitals that had or were scheduled to develop the capacity for open-heart surgery. But it also realized that the horse had already fled the barn; angiographic facilities, originally for diagnosis only but later proceeding to therapeutic interventions, had been operating for some time, without documented ill effect, in some Ontario hospitals lacking the capacity for open-heart surgery. In the absence of compelling evidence of poor results or accidents leading to death, and recognizing the increasing widespread demand for such services, the HSRC took the decision, somewhat reluctantly, not to advise the government against making the expenditures necessary to distribute both diagnostic and interventional angiography more broadly.

The other case relates to highly specialized pediatric care. Late in its mandate the commission established a task force, made up chiefly of representatives of

Ontario hospitals providing tertiary and quaternary care to children, to advise on whether to locate such facilities close to where patients and their families lived or to concentrate them in fewer hospitals with a critical mass of similar patients and subspecialist providers. There is increasing evidence that hospitals with heavy caseloads and more experienced specialists and nursing staff[9] have lower mortality rates for the same conditions than hospitals with fewer such patients (Kizer 2003). The trade-off between accessibility and quality, difficult for all patients, is particularly agonizing for children and their families. The pediatric literature had little to offer. After wrestling with the issue for months, the task force came down firmly on the side of retaining, indeed enhancing, sophisticated tertiary and quaternary services for children in all five of Ontario's Academic Health Science Centres (from which most of its members were drawn). This advice ran counter to the commissioners' intuition, so three highly experienced independent reviewers[10] (two of them pediatricians) were asked to review the report. They came to the diametrically opposite conclusion. They recommended that qualitative considerations be given priority over accessibility every time, and concluded that it was in the best interests of the children and their families to concentrate such services as open-heart surgery in one or both of Ontario's two superspecialized pediatric hospitals.

Since this conflicting advice came as the commission was nearing its sunset, the HSRC did not proceed with a recommendation to the ministry or with publication. Plainly, disrupting the status quo in pediatric quaternary care would be just too difficult politically for all concerned. Interestingly, financial considerations and the departure of the cardiac surgeon performing pediatric open-heart surgery drove University Hospital in London to close this service in 2003; patients requiring those procedures are now treated at the Hospital for Sick Children in Toronto or the Children's Hospital of Eastern Ontario in Ottawa. The issue has been revisited at least twice since the HSRC's sunset and was finally resolved when Premier McGuinty announced that pediatric cardiac surgery would be performed only at these two sites for the foreseeable future.

Two lessons can be learned from these experiences. The more esoteric and sophisticated the procedure, the higher the status of the institution and individuals who perform it; and the capacity for such work serves to attract health professionals, especially generalist and specialist physicians, to the hospital and community concerned.

Different people weigh the accessibility-versus-quality trade-off differently, especially as it applies to children and other vulnerable people and their families. Surely the best way to resolve such differences is to collect and widely distribute data on the outcomes of all interventions performed by health professionals and let truly informed patients and their families decide where and by whom they will be diagnosed and treated. After all, it is they who are at risk.

COMMUNICATION

Although it may have not been a lesson learned *de novo*, the need to proceed without perfect evidence was a lesson reinforced by the commission's having to base its decisions on no more than a fraction of the relevant information. There were two reasons for this deficiency. One was that, in many cases, while data were available they were incomplete or of questionable accuracy; the commission just did not have the time to verify them and fill in the blanks. At such times the commissioners and staff struggled to find a balance between thorough analysis and the paralysis engendered by endlessly repeating iterations of amended data sets, the robustness of which were suspect in the first place. The second reason for the deficiency was a lack of data bearing on many decisions that had to be made, especially those relating to community-based health care where records on the interactions between providers and users were sparse and not subject to the standards necessary to integrate them into intelligible databases. The inadequacy of Ontario's capacity for collecting, aggregating, sharing and managing health information, coupled with the need to "get on with things," drove the commission to take risks and to depend more on its own judgment and the advice of local experts than it would have done had harder evidence been available. Living with uncertainty gave the members of the HSRC a sense of what it must be like to work in the Ministry of Health (or in the government generally), answerable to the legislature for health care's huge budget. Without the substantial investment and "full-court press" needed to build capacity for health information management quickly, they and all Ontarians are sentenced to live with uncertainty for a long time to come.

The commission learned again and again, community by community, the importance of communicating — making people aware of the reason for change and keeping them informed about the process. Leadership is nothing without followers who are convinced, through good, honest communication, that their leaders are headed in the right direction.

Sorting between those who supported the commission and its objectives and those who did not was neither easy nor straightforward. A few organizations feigned neutrality while working assiduously behind the scenes, mainly within the ministry, to undermine and reduce the chances of the commission's recommendations, particularly those in phase II, from being implemented after its sunset. Some even masqueraded as supporters of at least parts of the HSRC's agenda, even to the point of speaking out in favour of certain initiatives, all the while biding their time until the commission was safely out of the way when they could bring their frank opposition out of the weeds. But these were in the minority. The great majority of organizations and individuals consulted by the commission, and those engaged in or affected by its work, were clear and open opponents or supporters of change and the HSRC's role in driving it.

NOTES

1. Attributed to R. Thompson, president of the Toronto Dominion Bank, circa 1995.
2. As distinct from decentralization, deconcentration and related organizational devices to bring the exercise of central power closer to those affected.
3. Although a few nominal networks remained in 2004, there were very few of the kind recommended by the HSRC, with combined, coordinated governance and management in common.
4. As given expression in the system of approving budgets by a series of separate "votes" in the House.
5. Notwithstanding the accompanying assurance that the total budget for health care would not be cut and the fact that the third of the scheduled cuts to the hospital envelope was not implemented.
6. The merger was strongly supported by the people in and around Cobourg and strenuously resisted by those in Port Hope, who later virtually boycotted the processes of planning and raising money for a new hospital.
7. A favourite remedy of one of Sinclair's mentors, Dr. E.H. Botterell.
8. See chapter 8, note 4.
9. See chapter 11.
10. Doctors Michel Bureau, Brian Postl and Charles Wright.

CHAPTER 11

IMPLICATIONS FOR PUBLIC POLICY

Ontario's approach — establishing and empowering the Health Services Restructuring Commission to restructure its public hospitals and advise it on strategies for restructuring everything else — differed substantially from the approaches to health care reform taken by other Canadian provinces beginning in the late 1990s. The Clair Commission in Quebec, the Fyke Commission in Saskatchewan and the Mazankowski Council in Alberta were comparable to the HSRC only in that they were advisory to government on what to do about the worsening problems in health care; unlike the HSRC, they had no power to direct. How effective was Ontario's unique approach?

Planning and scoping the capacity of the health-services system and its components is easier said than done. The development of public policy and plans to guide the evolution and growth of Canada's health services has challenged (and largely eluded) both provincial and federal health ministries. For instance, in recent times medical school enrolments and physician-to-population ratios have been decided nationally and implemented provincially, mainly on the basis of economic analyses (e.g., Barer and Stoddart 1991) and the recommendations of self-regulated colleges[1] on physician supply and demand, determined more or less unilaterally, without taking into account desirable (and actual) changes in the scope of practice of other health professionals. In Ontario, as hospital utilization patterns changed throughout the 1970s and 1980s, long-established bed-based planning parameters for hospitals became increasingly irrelevant. The advent of new utilization-management techniques, minimally invasive surgery, new pharmaceuticals and more comprehensive home-care alternatives to hospital care resulted in substantial changes to the use of hospital beds.

These were reinforced by marginal changes in funding policy made by the Ministry of Health to encourage hospitals to adopt new (and less costly) ways of doing business. The reduction in in-patient capacity in the late 1980s and early-to-mid-1990s was driven mainly by the application of fiscal levers designed to save money and in the absence of any plan outlining, in even general terms, how hospital capacity should be linked to the need for services. It was fortuitous that the benefits of technological innovation aligned with the financial pressures of the 1980s and 1990s to maintain service levels through the increasing use of safe and, in most cases, better community-based alternatives to in-patient care.

The culture or climate in terms of readiness for change is a critical factor in the implementation of organizational change. In complex organizations, typically the policies that drive successful change are set centrally while implementation of the initiatives and innovations takes place regionally or locally — as close as possible to the people affected.

When it created the HSRC in 1996, the government fell far short of setting the stage for change, of conditioning providers and, notwithstanding its relative readiness, the public for the magnitude of the changes that were about to take place. The culture of hospitals and other providers of health care presented many formidable barriers to change and a distinctly chilly climate. As we have seen, one condition the HSRC believed the government should have put in place was its vision of health care in Ontario or, at the least, a statement of its health care goals. In the absence of these tenets of planning, the HSRC was obliged to develop and disseminate its own vision and goals for a restructured health care system, so that those affected would be informed about the basis on which it was proceeding.

Similarly, the government did not provide the HSRC with a policy construct to guide its work. If such a construct existed, it was a well-kept secret. Nor did it provide a set of policies within which to determine the target capacities of hospitals and other components of the health care system and estimate the population's need for publicly insured or other health services. Accordingly, the commission had no option but to create its own policy framework, and quickly.

The health care world in Ontario and beyond was astonished by the speed with which the commission took charge, defined operating standards and filled the policy void within the government's bureaucracy. The framework knitted together a number of planning methodologies developed by consulting firms and academics to link past hospital utilization patterns, adjust for estimated growth and aging of the population, and incorporate the performance standards achieved by the top cluster of hospitals in the province. The HSRC also advised the government on policy, laying out explicitly the home and long-term-care capacity necessary to support a hospital sector reconfigured in accordance with its planning methodology. The planning parameters used, while as comprehensive as the data allowed, were nevertheless flawed by the assumption the commission had to accept (in the absence of an alternative) that past utilization was a reasonable proxy for need; there was no way to test the degree to which it also reflected available capacity (relative surplus or deficit), community by community. While the HSRC did its best with the data available, in retrospect, through its determination of hospital and community capacity, it should have been more aggressive in pushing for primary-care reform. By incorporating into its planning methodologies the fact that genuinely comprehensive primary-care services in every community would reduce the demand for hospital services, it might have stimulated the development and implementation of the bolder public policy necessary for more expeditious renewal of primary care throughout Ontario.

It remains, however, that for the first time the size of the hospital component of the system was estimated using a transparent method linking hospital capacity with that of home and long-term care. The HSRC's planning horizon expired in 2003 and no attempts have been made subsequently to update the framework or to set a new horizon. The policy vacuum with respect to the place of hospitals and their contributions to health care that pre-existed the commission appears to be re-emerging in 2004, a situation that will make it increasingly difficult for hospitals to plan for the future and will preclude integration of all the components necessary for a genuine health care system. Leadership disconnected from political considerations, as provided by the HSRC from 1996 to 2000, worked!

Why was such leadership effective in this case? Because the commission's mandate was clear, its authority was solidly based in legislation, it openly advertised the outcome it sought, the approaches it would take and the methods it would use, and it worked decisively and quickly. Notwithstanding the lack of a government-determined vision and policy framework, some 30 of Ontario's urban communities had recently debated the issues, and the reports of their District Health Councils (DHCs) had identified sensible decisions, at least in relation to hospital restructuring. Although in virtually every community, change elsewhere was preferable to change "here," there was widespread public recognition that change was needed or even long overdue. In addition, the new government had been elected with a strong majority on a platform of change. It was the "Common Sense Revolution." The time was ripe.

DEVOLUTION

A precondition for successful health care change is the capacity to implement it at a regional or local level. In 1996 the Ontario government had no structure in place to devolve health care decision-making to the communities affected. Although DHCs had been in place since the 1970s, they had never been well supported or given any real power. RHAs, structural mechanisms to exercise devolved authority for health services, have existed for 15 years in other provinces and longer in many other countries. In the United Kingdom, Sweden, Australia and New Zealand, geographic regions have long exercised considerable authority in the management and provision of health services and in some cases social services as well. In Canada, nine provinces have delegated to RHAs at least partial responsibility for the health of the population and the delivery of many health services. Their primary purpose is to consolidate the governance of many separate hospital and health agencies into one board, the RHA itself; another is to control escalating costs through better integration of services and to devolve to the regional entities some of the hard decisions regarding cuts and reforms. Some provincial governments have also given other health authorities province-wide responsibility for particular diseases/conditions such as mental health, cancer and cardiac care. The RHAs are responsible for managing hospitals, community health centres, home-care programs and a variety of long-term-care services. The expectation is that they will:

> ensure greater accountability by providers to the communities and taxpayers being served
> clarify the roles and responsibilities of all players, including providers, provider organizations and consumers
> differentiate the role of government, making clear its responsibility for system governance, central policy-making, setting standards and monitoring performance
> improve decision-making by linking resource allocation more directly with the needs of the population
> facilitate participation of consumer and other community groups in decision-making and ensure faster and more widely accepted responses to local community needs
> increase local, regional and central capacity for effective management of health information

> stimulate the development of reliable and valid measures, within each region, of accessibility, cost, quality of care and other measures of system performance, especially outcomes
> encourage the development of regional benchmarks to facilitate comparisons of regions within a province throughout a broad range of health indicators

These attempts to build capacity for change in the health care system have met with limited success. According to Lewis and Kouri (2004), RHAs have been able to consolidate programs at local and regional levels and there have been some successes in service integration. There are intersecting partnerships in place that may not have been possible without regionalization. The authors conclude that regionalization has resulted in less fragmentation of the system and less duplication of services in hospitals, and that admission to long-term residential care is now more streamlined and based more on need. It is clear that the goal of consolidation is being achieved; regionalization has brought a range of programs together under a single health authority and has disbanded a large number of sector-specific boards such as those for hospitals, nursing homes and home care.

Regionalization has fallen short of expectations, however, in a number of ways. First, there is no agreement on what the term really means and what scope of authority regional bodies should have. While the original expectation was that RHAs would truly take ownership of the health of regional populations, this has occurred only to a limited extent; the focus is still on service delivery. Also, in most provinces several important services such as those for drugs/pharmacare, mental health and cancer are outside the scope of RHAs. There has been very little attention to or investment in developing and managing health information, a deficiency that has severely restricted management capabilities and the accountability of RHAs (and central ministries). But perhaps the most significant deficiency is that RHAs have not been given any power over decisions concerning the payment of physicians, who continue to operate independently of them, or even over the rates of recompense of other health professionals and employees in institutions within their jurisdiction. As Lewis and Kouri point out, the attainment of health goals through regionalization depends on clear provincial commitments and explicitly devolved mandates. The provinces have wavered in their commitment to defined health goals and to the creation of policy frameworks for devolution, partly because they realize that, without appropriate measures and enhanced capacity for health information management, they cannot be held accountable, nor can RHAs be held accountable in any meaningful way for the achievement of defined goals and outcomes. All governments in Canada have proven vulnerable to pressures, mainly from the health care providers, to slow down the pace of reform, including reform through regionalization. As a politically viable alternative, they have tried to paper over the obvious problems with money — hence the continued growth in total health spending, well over the rate of inflation, between 1997 and 2005.

In the other provinces the devolution of authority to RHAs appears at first glance to have been radical and bold, but closer inspection reveals that it has been incremental and constrained. According to Lewis and Kouri, in some cases local programs and communities lost some of their original authority while governments retained more than met the eye; some have repatriated part of the authority previously devolved to the RHAs. Neither governments nor the public, much less health-service providers, seem ready to embrace fully the new regional entities and give them free rein to do what they have been set up to do. Everywhere devolution of authority has been incomplete; RHAs lack control over such important levers as recompense/incentive-setting and such significant and costly clinical programs as mental health and cancer services. Therefore, the objective evaluation of RHAs relative to Ontario's command-and-control approach to the governance and management of health care is not yet possible. Even in the event of true devolution of responsibility and authority to RHAs for the full range of health services, given the slow pace of change in health care the "regionalization experiment" would not yield to full evaluation for some years.

Ontario has been referred to, tongue in cheek, as Canada's control group — the sole province not to implement regionalization.[2] The control is somewhat contaminated, however! Ontario's DHCs, which had responsibility for district/regional planning for over two decades, had completed a good deal of work on restructuring hospital and other services in their communities before the HSRC arrived on the scene. Regrettably, the government did not pull together the best practices from this work as the basis for its development of a common set of policies on restructuring. A set of conclusions from the work of DHCs in relation to mental health care, rehabilitation and long-term care would have been of real benefit to the commission with regard to what standards and operating principles to apply to its decisions on hospital restructuring and its recommendations on reinvestments in community-based services. In retrospect, the commission itself could and should have done more to engage the DHCs in accelerating the pace of its work. As it was, the DHCs were left to float freely, relatively disconnected from the HSRC. At the same time, the government began to reduce their number from over 30 to 17, and by the end of the commission's mandate the ministry was about to decentralize itself into seven provincial planning regions. All this contributed to the DHCs' uncertainty about their role and scope and their sense of being underused and undervalued.

Prior to the commission's formation, the issue of devolution had been the subject of public-policy debate for over three decades. In various forms and using different terms — decentralization, deconcentration, devolution, regionalization, network formation — many policy advisers and planners had recommended the redistribution of responsibility, authority and accountability for the management of health and social services, and some aspects of their governance as well, to regional/local decision-makers. Although Ontario was criticized for failing to implement regionalization, as all the other provinces had done, in fact its establishment of the HSRC in 1996, with its power to restructure the province's public hospitals, constituted Canada's truest and boldest experiment with devolution. The unprecedented conferring of power to order hospitals to close, amalgamate, transfer or accept programs, change volumes and so on startled health-policy critics. Previously, successive Ontario governments had established arm's-length commissions, councils, agencies, task forces and the like (including the DHCs) to advise on how best to reform health care in all its aspects, but none had delegated the authority to actually effect change. The extent of the commission's power over hospitals was truly remarkable; approved by the legislature, it was binding even on the minister and the Ministry of Health — the government itself. The only constraint was that its power of decision had to be exercised fairly and with a view to serving the public interest.

In addition to the devolution of real power, Ontario's experiment in devolution — the HSRC — differed from regionalization in the other provinces in that it did not have as a goal the takeover of hospital boards. Whereas most health authorities consolidated the governance of the hospitals, home-care agencies, nursing homes and some other provider organizations in their regions "to overcome the atomization of the system," as Lewis and Kouri put it, the HSRC did not. Whereas RHAs take direct responsibility for the provision of selected health services, the commission was never intended to play an operational role. Although the HSRC did order the consolidation of a number of hospital boards, it respected the fundamental concept that the governance and management of hospitals (and other institutions and organizations providing health services to a community, district or region) remain in the hands of the populations they serve, separate from government and its agencies, the single major "purchasers" of hospital and other health services.

As well as demonstrating the effectiveness of devolved authority in leading such powerful elements of the health care system as hospitals, home care and long-term care and in filling, however imperfectly, the policy vacuum, the HSRC proved to be a remarkably effective catalyst for change. One reason for the commission's effectiveness was the fact that it did not dismantle the existing governing structures but worked through them, especially hospital boards, collectively one of the largest, most organized and most powerful players in the health care system. Making change quickly and successfully in hospitals, the system's big spenders, with their power, influence and long-established ability to "work the system," served as a salutary example to others.

GETTING THINGS DONE

The commission's effectiveness was also well served by its early decision to work hard and fast — to achieve as much as possible before the government pulled the rug from under it. Several lessons apply. First, it was vital that the HSRC make it clear that it had the authority to take action, not just to recommend that others (i.e., the government) do so. Second, the commission's open development of its vision for the future of Ontario's health system served to avoid surprising those affected by its decisions; in leading the way to change, it mapped out a path for others to follow. Third, despite the absence of government standards, the commission was able to set population-health criteria, standards and utilization guidelines with a view to ensuring fair and equitable access to hospital and other health services throughout the province. The "man in the moon test" — every decision had to make sense — was a key factor. And, vitally important, with politics removed from the decision-making process, the rules of the game were transparent.

What other lessons bearing on health policy can public policy-makers draw from the experience of Ontario's Health Services Restructuring Commission? Established to do a specific job — to restructure public hospitals and advise government on other changes necessary to foster the development of a true health care system — the commission came up against policy issues at every turn. In some cases existing policy was obstructionist. On example was the government's slavish adherence to the legislative vote system that cements the allocation of funds to specific purposes; this was alleged to disallow consolidation of the provincial funding of mental health services into envelopes to be managed regionally by local stakeholders. And there was a marked lack of interest in even considering the articulation of an ideal health care system for Ontario, much less developing a coherent policy framework to achieve it.

As we enter the twenty-first century, how might the HSRC experience apply to the development of a contemporary policy framework for the delivery of health services in Ontario and throughout Canada? It is obvious that considerable change is necessary in many aspects of health care. It is also obvious that there is consensus not only on the need for change but also on its general direction. It is fair to say that, collectively, the conclusions of the HSRC in Ontario, the Clair Commission in Quebec, the Fyke Commission in Saskatchewan, the Mazankowski Council in Alberta and, nationally, the Standing Senate Committee on Social Affairs, Science and Technology and the Romanow Royal Commission show clear consensus on the majority of those changes (there remain differences to resolve, but these relate primarily to strategies and tactics, not to policy):

> Universally available publicly funded insurance should continue to be the bedrock of health care throughout Canada.
> The publicly funded system must be made both sustainable and affordable by some combination of greater productivity and new funding arrangements.
> Health care must be made more comprehensive through the extension of its coverage to a range of "medically necessary" services such as home care, especially for post-hospital patients and those in need of palliative care, and to catastrophic drug costs. Medical necessity is in itself a poor definition of comprehensiveness.
> There must be greater accountability, on the part of governments to their citizens and on the part of the system to taxpayers and governments, in relation to health outcomes (return on expenditures) and to patients and their families for their timely access to services, the quality of services they receive and, above all, their health outcomes.
> The health care system must be made more real. It is essential that vulnerable people and their families be provided with continuity of care — smoother coordination and integration of the work of the many service providers.

> The governance and management of health care must be "beefed up." There is a leadership vacuum to fill. Governments need to govern, to provide policy direction and funding and devolve to those closer to the people affected the responsibility for organizing and managing health-service providers and allocating funding appropriate to their contributions.
> The first step is to transform primary care, creating multidisciplinary teams of health professionals to provide a range of comprehensive services 24 hours a day, 7 days a week. This must be combined with a shift in incentives to achieve a better balance between care for the sick and health promotion/disease prevention.
> A consistent, more long-range policy perspective is essential with regard to the education, training, certification (and recertification) of doctors, nurses and other health professionals, their interrelationships and the scope of their practices.
> Hospital-based care should be increasingly rationalized, through application of the principles of critical mass and the Clair Commission's "hierarchy of sophistication," to safeguard its quality and cost-effectiveness.
> High priority should be given to greatly enhancing the capacity of health information management. This is key to the development of the set of policies needed to achieve many if not all of the other health-care changes.

One of the urgent challenges faced by the commission relates to the leadership vacuum referred to above — the lack of effective governance of the health care system. The HSRC did not fully appreciate the thinness of the policy framework in place to support decision-making in health care until it began its work; then it realized that there were few planning guidelines for hospital restructuring and the sectors that it would affect, such as home and long-term care. Given the need to proceed quickly, the commission had to conduct its own research in order to address the potential impact of its decisions and recommendations on, for example, the governance of hospitals and their human resources, including physicians with privileges. The development of the vision for a future health care system required broad consultation, a necessary step in creating the context for change. The development of reinvestment guidelines led to policy questions relating to:

> expansion of home-care capacity and raising of the profile of home care, in particular the potential of short-term home care to ease the burden of ALC patients on hospitals and meet the needs of acute-care patients equally well and much less expensively

> the need for some 20,000 additional long-term-care places in Ontario
> divestment of the ownership and management of Provincial Psychiatric Hospitals, a policy issue central to the elimination of discrimination and stigma with regard to people with mental illness
> the associated implementation of mental health planning guidelines (30 beds/100,000 population) developed in the early 1990s but never implemented
> a method for estimating the ongoing need for mental health beds/capacity for children and adolescents and benchmarks for their equitable distribution throughout Ontario
> improved planning of formal networks and coordination or integration of, for example, rehabilitation, pediatric and French-language services
> estimation of the need for capital investment to support restructuring and expansion in the hospital and long-term-care sectors

No organization or collection of disparate services such as the health care system requires can function or evolve without decisive leadership based on a shared vision. Perhaps the most significant single contribution of Ontario's Health Services Restructuring Commission was its demonstration of effective leadership. By articulating its vision for the future and filling the policy vacuum, the commission played a role more properly played, in a democracy, by government. The many changes made during and immediately following the commission's work clearly show the importance of decisive leadership, policy direction and expeditious decision-making. This is the role of Canada's provincial and territorial governments, the entities responsible for ensuring the effective collaboration of the many individuals, organizations and institutions that together provide the services needed to optimize the health of the population. If political considerations prevent governments from running their health care systems, one option is to do as the Ontario government did in 1996, and as suggested more recently by a former premier, Bob Rae: devolve the responsibility and authority to an arm's-length body (Rae's comments are elaborated below). This course of action would not serve the interests of democracy over the long term, but it could be effective in the short term, or as long as it took to refocus bureaucracies and build their capacity to support governance instead of management and, equally important, to create mechanisms for insulating governments against political influence on day-to-day governance decisions. Clearly, governments must continue to be held accountable for their decisions, including those related to health care, but in aggregate, at election time, not, as tends to be the case now, on a decision-by-decision basis.

The HSRC's arm's-length position did distance the minister and government from the political consequences of the commission's individual decisions. But it did not and could not insulate them from the collective political consequences of its actions, which, in any case, proved not to diminish the Harris Conservatives' chances of being re-elected.

Less obvious is how health care's public-policy practitioners are to remake successfully or construct *de novo* the policy framework in place over the past 40 years to meet the challenges of the twenty-first century. It is one thing to know what to do, quite another to find ways of making the necessary changes within the political, financial and other constraints that apply in health care. What lessons from the processes, findings and outcomes of the HSRC apply to this change process regionally, provincially and nationally?

There is no doubt that health care is a sticky issue — resistant, slow and hard to change. To some extent that is a good thing: it minimizes the incidence of serious mistakes caused by expedient, spur-of-the-moment decisions. But the sluggishness of the last decade has been extreme. It constitutes a far greater danger to health care in Canada than the changes recommended by the HSRC and other provincial and national bodies.

The HSRC's experience demonstrates that health care can be changed successfully — and quickly. The commission's leadership did not please everyone, but it was effective. Half a decade later, those affected are, with few exceptions, striving to go forward, as evidenced by the restructured subsystems of urban public hospitals and the provincial investment in community services, primarily home and long-term care.

While conventional wisdom holds that change in public services is best made slowly and in small steps, the HSRC's bold, big-bang approach was clearly effective; as a means of achieving change in health care, it is a practical alternative to incrementalism, pilot projects and the like. This is not a new observation. The introduction of publicly funded insurance to cover physicians' services in 1962 is a case in point. Ironically the doctors' strike in Saskatchewan would now almost certainly be replicated, and be much more prolonged and bitter, if the policy were reversed and physicians' services "delisted." In the introduction to their report, Michel Clair and his colleagues propose that Quebec engage in "a sort of 'big bang' of ideas and ways of looking at things" followed by a three-year period in which the entire health and social services system would "evolve toward" the vision established. A three-year evolutionary process would be an extraordinarily short one given the current rate of change in health care. The Clair report does acknowledge, however, that gradual implementation will make it easier for government to find the funding to create the conditions needed to "induce the principal players involved to...adopt the direction of change" — in other words, to reward those who embrace the recommended changes and penalize those who resist them (Commission d'étude sur les services de santé et les services sociaux 2001, vi, 228).

While gradual implementation has the advantage of the time and experience needed to get the players onside, it also offers the gift of time to those opposed to change. The slow pace of implementing even watered-down models of primary-care reform in Ontario, the outcome of negotiations between the Ontario Medical Association and the government, is a case in point. To illustrate further, it was agreed in the mid-1990s that the fee schedule for the Ontario Health Insurance Program should be brought up to date to reflect cumulative changes, over many years, in knowledge, technology and practices. The joint OMA/Ministry of Health Resource Based Relative Value Commission, chaired by Dr. John Wade,[3] was struck in 1997 with a mandate to create a complete and indivisible relative value fee schedule. Its report, not completed until 2002, recommended many changes to reflect the development of new knowledge, the availability of technology, and recompense of family physicians and other specialists based on their training, skills and levels of responsibility (Resource Based Relative Value Commission 2002). The changes were opposed by those specialists, led by ophthalmologists, radiologists and others, whose incomes might be lowered and, through the associated changes in incentives, whose power and influence might be weakened. The report sank without a trace. Unprepared to impose on physicians and others either a fair and modern fee schedule or new forms of practice organization — primary care is the key example — the Ontario government seems to have lost control of the alternative lever of negotiating changes in the incentive structure to achieve greater health care productivity, at least on the part of physicians.

Implementation of the restructuring of urban hospitals ordered by the HSRC is still a work in progress several years after the commission closed its doors. Yet following the commission's establishment in 1996 the overall policy framework for hospital restructuring, based on the work of the DHCs, was, with few exceptions, measured in months. Hospital consolidation based on that framework would not have continued without the commission's having the power to order hospital restructuring and the determination to use that power quickly. Even with the firm, committed direction provided to Ontario's hospitals, planning and effecting the changes has been a slow process, extending well beyond the usual time horizons of governments.

In addition to the commission's determination to preserve or enhance the accessibility, quality and affordability (cost-effectiveness) of hospital-based services, the policy that guided its decisions was that of critical mass — the principle that those who do things frequently achieve better outcomes than those who do them infrequently. Although relatively thin at the time, evidence bearing on the applicability of this principle to health services, especially hospital-based services, has appeared in the literature in recent years (e.g., Birkmeyer et al. 2002, 2003; Finlayson, Goodney and Birkmeyer 2003; Kizer 2003).

This critical-mass principle was also applied by the Clair and Fyke Commissions and the Mazankowski Council in supporting their recommendations that hospitals be sharply differentiated in terms of the sophistication of their services and be organized into what the Clair report refers to as a hierarchy. It is also a feature of the report and recommendations of the Standing Senate Committee. Notwithstanding the inequity of access created if there were, for example, few hospitals in the country offering pediatric open-heart surgery, it was the view of every provincial commission that the safeguard of better outcomes should prevail following the aggregation of skilled personnel and facilities into a critical or optimum mass in those few hospitals. Right of access is an empty right indeed if it is to a hospital-based service that is not of the highest possible quality and puts a successful outcome at greater risk than would an alternative, larger hospital more specialized in that particular service, even if distant from the patient's home and family.

The first lesson bearing on health-policy development to be drawn from the work of the HSRC relates to the policy of devolution — government's assignment of health care decisions to arm's-length bodies. Ironically it is in the province that, until recently, constituted Canada's control group for regionalization that the most independent power and authority have ever been devolved. In contrast to the advisory bodies set up in Quebec, Saskatchewan and Alberta, Ontario's HSRC was given real power — the power to restructure public hospitals. The results so far show that the actions taken on the HSRC's directions and on its recommendation of massive reinvestment in the capacity of community-based care have been much more extensive and rapid than those taken elsewhere. Given the painfully slow pace of change in health care, however, it remains to be seen which of the four provincial bodies will have the greatest effect as reflected in implementation of its recommendations. Recently the four chairs, optimists at heart, had occasion to compare the results to date. They expressed frustration at the slow pace of action taken on the recommendations that each body had been convinced, on the strength of both available evidence and expert opinion, represented the best and most viable means of preserving and enhancing health care in its province. All four men, two of whom had extensive political experience,[4] identified the chief roadblock as a lack of political will to "take on" those who resist change, principally organized medicine, public sector unions and the representatives of small community hospitals fearing the loss of their autonomy.

In the spring of 2004 Bob Rae, speaking at the Canadian Club in Kingston about the large and growing opportunity cost of health care, was asked what he would do to constrain and reform the "800-pound gorilla" were he to be premier again. Rae replied that he believed governments per se are incapable of reforming health care, the political imperative of re-election being too powerful and interest-consuming (as demonstrated by the withdrawal by the Harris government of the HSRC's powers as the 1999 election approached). He said he would set up an arm's-length body akin to the HSRC and reminiscent of the Ontario Hospital Services Commission, established many years ago when publicly funded hospital insurance was introduced in the province, and give it the much broader mandate of changing the entire health care system in accordance with a policy framework developed by government. His suggested priorities were a focus on primary care and much expanded home and long-term care co-ordinated with hospital-based care (the HSRC's first priority would have been building the capacity for health information management). Although never formally recommended to the Ontario government, the concept of re-creating the Hospital Services Commission but with a mandate encompassing health services broadly was the subject of a number of unofficial discussions within the HSRC. The commissioners conceived the membership of this hypothetical body as being appointed by the government, which would, in any event, inherit any and all political consequences flowing from its actions. There is debate, of course, about how the delegation of such politically sensitive decision-making would sit with the tradition of parliamentary democracy, but no government can or should escape the political ramifications of its decisions, whether made internally or by a body to which it had delegated the requisite authority.

The HSRC experience in Ontario demonstrates that the single lever of funding allocation is insufficient, in the hands of government, to steer the provider/constituents of such a complex system as health care toward the desired outcomes. It is a lever best used locally as a management tool at the workface, as a complement to the more powerful forces available to governments: leadership in the realization of a vision; the setting of goals and objectives; policy direction embedded in legislation, enforceable by law; evaluation of performance and outcomes; and, in the end, the authority of the electorate to speak and act on its behalf.

There has been a good deal of discussion, especially in relation to RHAs, about the selection of membership of bodies to which governments may devolve responsibility and authority. The fact that the HSRC was established under the terms of an act of the legislature signalled that its authority was not subject to the direction or even the influence of the government. As discussed previously, this was central to decisions made by the courts when the commission's directions were challenged. Nevertheless, the HSRC's members were appointed by the cabinet[5] according to the principle that governments appoint at least a majority of the members of bodies charged with making decisions for which the government of the day will bear political responsibility. There are some indications from other jurisdictions that election by local constituencies of members of, for example, RHAs, has functioned poorly if at all. One reason for this result has been the difficulty in finding community leaders willing to stand for election. Another is the concern that a locally elected authority will become just another advocacy body unprepared to face hard decisions at that level, preferring to shunt difficult issues to the ministry concerned using the excuse "You didn't give us enough money"; Lewis and Kouri note that this concern is expressed by government officials while RHAs themselves believe they stand up well against local pressures (2004). The commission's experience shows that regardless of how the members of arm's-length bodies are selected and appointed, it is vital that they be free of government influence in their decision-making and completely immune from political considerations and lobbying by local or other interests.

BARRIERS TO CHANGE

First among the barriers to the HSRC's recommended changes was the government's lack of political courage and will as the commission grew more comfortable in its mandate (especially in its second phase) to confront three forces:

> the members of caucus from key constituencies (then northern and rural Ontario communities with small hospitals eager to retain their autonomy), with their deeply vested local interests and strong supporters with connections, especially in the media
> organized health professionals, including physicians (OMA) and nurses (Ontario Nurses Association, Registered Nurses Association of Ontario), the Ontario Hospital Association and public sector unions, each group with its well-financed and well-staffed capacity for influencing public opinion through the media — and sometimes through messages communicated directly to patients and their families in physicians' offices or by individual practitioners
> deeply vested bureaucratic interests within the government itself. The Ministry of Health did not welcome the prospect of exchanging the minutiae of micromanagement and the rush associated with being lobbied by powerful people for a focus on policy development and governance issues. Within the organization those concerned with policy are known to have much lower status than their counterparts in the more operational branches. Compounding the fear of change was creeping emasculation of the ministry by the overcentralization in the Management Board and the premier's office of important decision-making, especially that related to policy matters, no matter how small. With devolution of their management responsibilities, many ministry bureaucrats feared they would have no role (or jobs) at all!

The principal barrier, though, was the unwillingness or inability of governments to take the case for change directly to the public. In the struggle for the support of public opinion, "death in the street" rhetoric and exaggerated anecdotes recounted by hired opinion-makers will usually carry the day, a fact well known to the organizations representing health professionals, hospitals and their employees, and other providers of health services. The system's capacity for health information management is just not up to the task of bringing to bear much in the way of objective evidence on issues that may be in dispute, such as the productivity of health professionals (few measures of outcomes exist) or waiting times (apart from the Cardiac Care Network and a few others being developed, no criteria-ordered waiting lists are available for public scrutiny in Ontario). Lacking credible evidence, governments are easily outgunned on the public stage by the well-oiled and well-financed public relations machinery of health-provider organizations.

Governments' lack of success in the public-opinion wars is compounded by the fact that the credibility of politicians, bureaucrats and governments themselves is so much lower than that of doctors, nurses and just about everybody, certainly all those connected with the provision of health services. Interestingly, the HSRC appeared not to be tarred with the same brush. Its communications strategy included taking its case directly to the public as vigorously as it could, mainly through the media, presenting evidence when it could and openly arguing opinions when it could not. It is difficult to assess the result, but it is a matter of record that as the hospital restructuring phase of the commission's work wound down — a phase that saw an unprecedented amount of change in Ontario's urban hospitals within a short period — the government went to the polls and was re-elected with a large majority. The HSRC's leadership of change in health care — decisive, apolitical and transparent — was not a political liability; indeed it may well have been an asset.

Finally, a significant barrier was the fact that the Ontario government lacked the financial resources necessary to implement many of the HSRC's recommended strategies. It may have been able to overcome that barrier by changing its priorities in relation to tax cuts and the rate of deficit reduction, but funds remained in very short supply throughout the period 1996-2000. The large increments in health care funding by both levels of government in recent years, following the financial downturn of the early to mid-1990s, have at best alleviated the system's growing problems — papered them over, as Lewis and Kouri put it; they are in more urgent need of fixing now than they were in 2000. The case can be made that more money has had a paradoxical effect on health care. Perhaps what is needed to foster the fundamental changes that successive provincial and national bodies, including the HSRC, have called for is a financial crisis so dire and prolonged that even those with deeply vested interests in the status quo will demand them.

Practically, though, there are only two reasons why people change — they will be better off if they do (the carrot), or they will be worse off if they don't (the stick) — and carrots beat sticks every time. It *will* cost money to "buy change," to rebuild and to purchase or build new capital resources, structures, technology and infrastructure. But the major investment needed is in changing the incentives in the system, in rewarding increases in productivity — the outcomes measured in terms of better health of individuals and the population for the vast sums spent on health care. Given that at least 75 percent of health care costs go to pay people, greater productivity and cost-effectiveness can be achieved without threat to the quality of care only if the substitution of lower-cost for higher-cost labour is encouraged, as has been the practice in virtually all other sectors of the economy for many years. Research, training, continuing education and skills development have been used in many countries to support the substitution of physician assistants, nurses and nurse practitioners for physicians, for example, or of nurse anaesthetists for anesthesiologists and technical assistants and coaches for physical therapists. If providers of primary care were paid on the basis of their impact on the health of the populations they serve (outcomes), combined with measures of "customer satisfaction," rather than the rate of throughput for which fee-for-service currently provides such a strong incentive, substantial improvement in the productivity of primary care would soon result. Such changes in incentive structures would not in themselves cost much money — over the long term, in fact, they would reduce costs through the productivity gains achieved. But the new ways of doing business in health care would have to be supported by two financial investments:

> new capital structures, such as purpose-built primary-care facilities and expansion of the specialized facilities necessary for a hierarchical array of hospitals to concentrate their efforts on the particular surgical and other services most needed in their catchments

> rapid expansion of the system's capacity for health information management, an imperative for genuine health care reform throughout the country

Since the commission closed its doors in 2000, there have been some changes in the policy environment. The Canadian economy has improved; most governments now have balanced budgets and the overall debt-to-GDP ratio is shrinking. But, perhaps as a result of what are seen to be better times, the impetus for change has dissipated, notwithstanding the fact that a large structural deficit remains and most provinces continue to experience financial stress. With respect to health care, in the latter part of the 1990s the focus was on systemic change as the way to resolve its problems, but now "underfunding" is once again the issue. Most troubling of all, public confidence in the system continues to erode under the pressure of lengthening waiting lists, fewer family physicians in remote, rural and small-town Canada, continuing media reports of physician shortages and waiting times, and the "hard times" rhetoric of health care providers and workers. All of this is compounded by highly publicized wrangling between Ottawa and the provinces and territories over who should take how much responsibility for spending more of the Canadian taxpayer's dollars on health care.

The most important lesson to be taken from the experience of Ontario's Health Services Restructuring Commission is that health information management is key. Those responsible for the governance of the system — and effective governance is vital — must have at their disposal a wealth of information on the myriad individual interactions between providers and consumers of health care and their outcomes, comparable to that available for the banking system and most other sectors of the economy. Such information is essential to inform the public policies needed in order to establish a health care system that will meet the needs of Canadians into the future. It is also essential that the public be provided with accountability for the use of their considerable tax (and private) contributions.

Creating the required capacity for health information management will not be cheap; the HSRC estimated that $500 to $700 million over three years was needed in Ontario alone to establish effective governance of a health information management system and lay the foundation for its development. But information management is the single most important factor in changing the status quo, in making the changes needed to establish the high-quality, sustainable health care system that people want and should expect to have wherever they live and work in Canada. As for the cost of that system, only with a functional health information management system can the legitimate question "Are we getting our money's worth?" be answered. So far, the only possible answer is "Who knows?" And with a total annual expenditure in excess of $130 billion that is just not good enough.

The commissioners and personnel who lived this story of Ontario's Health Services Restructuring Commission between 1996 and 2000 had the great privilege of participating in a bold experiment to move the health care mountain. They have shown that health care's inertia *can* be overcome. The challenge now is to build on the momentum generated by the commission, to continue and accelerate the work in progress in order to create a genuinely accessible, affordable system that guarantees the availability of high-quality health services to those who need them. The challenge is to take that second step to "reorganize and revamp the delivery system...the big thing we haven't done yet."

NOTES

1. The Ontario College of Family Physicians and the Royal College of Physicians and Surgeons of Canada.
2. In September 2004 the Ontario Ministry of Health announced its decision to devolve some decision-making responsibility (and authority over funding allocations) to bodies referred to as Local Health Integration Networks (LHINs) – regionalization, perhaps, by another name. Unlike regionalization elsewhere, however, the intention is not to consolidate hospital, CCAC and other boards; such local boards are to retain governance responsibility for the services their institution or organization provides, while the LHIN is to allocate funding and ensure the coordination of all health services. The purpose is to foster system integration and clearer accountability of provider organizations, individually and collectively.
3. A former dean of medicine at the University of Manitoba and later deputy minister of health in Manitoba.
4. Don Mazankowski and Michel Clair.
5. Through individual orders-in-council.

AFTERWORD: TOWARD A GENUINE HEALTH CARE SYSTEM

Following on Tommy Douglas's remarks in 1982, it is encouraging to see policy initiatives finally emerging to foster the creation of genuine health care systems in Canada. If not pan-Canadian, very similar systems for the delivery of health care are becoming recognizable, province by province. All of them represent, with some minor differences, increasing organization/revamping of the delivery of care. It is clear that both levels of government, federal and provincial/territorial, have come to see that Douglas's second step is vital to the future of what Canadians know as medicare. That second step must be taken — and soon.

Yet the trajectory of system building continues to be distressingly flat. In addition to the political challenge of change, many key policy issues have yet to be discussed, much less settled, by the governments that must take responsibility for governing our health care system.

Perhaps the most important of these policy issues has to do with vision — what a real system of health care, or, better yet, of health *and* health care, should look like in the twenty-first century. In the mid-twentieth century the vision was to provide Canadians with universal access to hospital and physician services without undue risk to their personal financial resources. Publicly funded insurance was the instrument that, as Premier Douglas put it, removed the financial barrier between those who needed health services and those who provided them.

Since then much has changed. We now recognize the powerful effects of many factors, in addition to health services, on the health of individuals and of the population. It is increasingly obvious that people need many health services, in addition to those provided in hospital and by physicians, to recover from illness and injury and to maintain their health.

Taking the optimistic view that our governments have finally grasped the nettle and have decided that we are to organize a real system of health care delivery, a key policy question is how broad in scope it should be. Should the purpose of the system be to ensure universal access but to a wider range of services? If it is, we will have to decide on the size of the "medicare basket" and on the process of determining what goes into it. Or should the purpose of the system be to aim higher — to optimize the health of the population?

Most Canadians would agree that the system should both meet individual care needs *and* promote population health. That dual purpose should be clearly set out and our health care systems structured and funded accordingly, keeping in mind the opportunity costs imposed by the everpresent resource limits on the achievement of both objectives. Health services are fairly readily defined, but where should all those other public services that affect the health of populations begin and end, in terms of their inclusion or exclusion from the publicly funded system?

Given the political, financial and cultural realities of Canada and the countries with which we compare ourselves, it is unrealistic to conceive of extending the principle of publicly funded insurance across the whole spectrum of services that bear on the health of the population. The spectacular failure of centrally planned economies like that of the Soviet Union to develop and operate health-optimizing systems illustrates the futility of taking that path. Even if it were possible, Canadians have no political appetite for a "nanny state" in their lives, even if it were to increase their lifespans by a year or two.

But putting aside the notion of everything being 100 percent publicly funded, one can easily conceive of a real system of health care, one that offers both improved comprehensive sickness care and services designed to optimize the health of the population. The current system includes public health services and other programs intended to prevent disease and promote health. Some elements (hospital and physician care and many public health services) are exclusively publicly funded, others (such as dentistry and nonprescription drugs) are almost entirely privately funded and most of those in the category of comprehensive health services are funded by a public-private mixture. Arguments will never end about the ideal balance between public and private funding,[1] but it is a fact that significant private payment, either directly or through supplementary insurance offered by the private sector, will continue to feature in the financing of such services in Canada.

It is also a fact that the evolving system of health care delivery in Canada's provinces and territories will remain partly in the hands of providers who are in the private sector, legally and practically. Only in a nightmare could one conceive of a system that is totally publicly owned and operated, one in which all health professionals — physicians, pharmacists, dentists, therapists, providers of long-term and home care, and so on — are public servants. One of the "zombies" (bad ideas that never die [Barer 2005]) referred to by health-policy people is the notion that the *Canada Health Act*'s fifth principle of public administration applies to the provision of health care by physicians and in hospital. In fact, the fifth principle applies only to administration of the provincial/territorial programs of publicly funded health insurance under medicare.

Much has been made of the announcement of plans to transform health care delivery in Alberta by adopting a "third way," "drawing on the experiences and best ideas from other health care systems, both elsewhere in Canada and around the world." Premier Ralph Klein is quoted as saying:

> The Third Way is about being open to new ideas to meet the needs of patients within the context of the Canada Health Act. It has to get us beyond the endless, pointless debates about private versus public health care and recognize that privately delivered health care is just one more option for delivering health care services. (Alberta Health and Wellness 2005)

Many have decoded the word "private" in this context to mean extending the for-profit concept beyond physicians to privately owned hospitals competing with the not-for-profit hospitals governed by Alberta's Regional Health Authorities (RHAs). If that is the intention, it is but a small perturbation of the status quo in Alberta and elsewhere in Canada, where for-profit and not-for-profit nursing homes, diagnostic laboratories and home-care agencies have for many years competed for patients/clients. As with significant funding derived from private spending, both directly out-of-pocket and through supplementary insurance, the "private" provision of virtually all services should and will continue to be a feature of Canadian health care.

Neither the "private" provision of the spectrum of health services nor the present admixture of funding derived from both the public and private purses is inconsistent with the development of a genuine health care system for Canada. But the development and successful operation of such a system depends on strong leadership. Governments will have to provide effective governance, policy direction and a range of incentives derived from public funding, combined with regulations based in legislation, to ensure the wholehearted participation of all parties in realizing the vision of a system.

Democracy's foundation rests on an informed citizenry's confidence in its elected leaders. Despite the enormous sums of money involved, without a consensual vision of a health care system appropriate to their present and anticipated needs, Canadians are not sufficiently informed about how their money, public or private, is being spent. How can they judge the appropriateness and quality of their political leadership if they do not know where their leaders are headed? The absence of a contemporary vision of health and health care represents an enormous policy vacuum, federally and provincially, that will continue to stifle reform efforts. Health care has to be about more than waiting lists, troublesome as these are.

Another important policy issue relates to the public funding of health insurance. The arcane arguments about how the two senior levels of government should share the credit and blame for raising and spending taxpayers' money on health insurance should be refocused on a more fundamental question: whether there are better ways of raising revenue than the current model of funding the costs out of general taxation (supplemented in some provinces by consumption taxes and income-tested premiums treated more or less as taxes).

When publicly funded insurance for medical services was initiated in Canada, it was intended that consumers be responsible for a proportion of the health care costs they incur (Kent 2000). The idea was that this would be an incentive for people to avoid behaviours that put their health at risk, to embrace preventive care and to refrain from seeking professional attention for trivial matters. The idea of reintroducing user fees at the point of service keeps cropping up. However, it is well known that they deter poor people with numerous health problems from seeking professional assistance and do not deter consumers with very minor problems from doing so; they too have been dubbed a "zombie." Yet user fees/copayments continue to be a feature in all health services except for those provided by physicians and in hospitals under medicare.[2] Notwithstanding medicare's first-dollar coverage, it is generally agreed that significant benefits could be derived from the introduction of supplemental funding in order to raise awareness among users and providers alike about the costs of health services and to improve accountability — providing a foundation for the determination of cost-benefit ratios. To that end, the much-discussed concept of medical savings accounts (Gratzer 1999; Forget, Deber and Roos 2002) was proposed by the

Mazankowski Council in Alberta (Mazankowski 2001), although not as a supplement to general taxation.

In its comprehensive report on health care in Canada, the Standing Senate Committee on Social Affairs, Science and Technology recommends the development of a hypothecated tax to fund its proposed program of publicly funded insurance against catastrophic drug costs (2002b). Other proposals for raising supplemental funds for public health care and for increasing accountability have more general application. One such proposal is for a copayment or variable-premium health insurance program, based on the user-pay principle and administered through the personal income tax system (Aba, Goodman and Mintz 2002). The rationale is that a proportion (40 percent) of the public expenditures on health care made on a person's behalf should be regarded as a basic consumption expenditure, akin to food and shelter, and be reimbursed to the government; the reimbursement would be subject both to an exemption below a floor level of family income (e.g., $10,000) and to an upper limit of 3 percent of annual income. A proposal by Tom Kent, one of the fathers of medicare, is to increase revenues by treating health services received by individuals as a taxable benefit in the calculation of personal income tax, with an annual upper limit to insure against catastrophic costs and exemption for those with little or no taxable income (Aba, Goodman and Mintz 2002).

A closely related issue is the share of health care costs that are appropriately borne by the state and the individuals who receive the care. Currently, with a roughly 70/30 percent public/private split for the spectrum of health services, broadly defined, Canada ranks low among OECD countries, considerably higher (in terms of the public share) than the United States but with more reliance on out-of-pocket and private insurance funding than most other countries. Despite the fact that user charges and copayments were a feature of medicare at the outset, the Romanow Commission and others (Royal Commission on the Future of Health Care in Canada 2002) have articulated the view that "the notion that use of health care services would become an economic decision for individuals rather than something they simply use when they have a felt need is…against the grain of what has become, for good or ill, a value judgment held by many Canadians" (Rode and Rushton 2002, 4).

Yet the most recent first ministers' health accords and the reports of the Standing Senate Committee and the Romanow Commission all reflect an extraordinary logical inconsistency. They reject any reconsideration of the now almost iconic principle in the *Canada Health Act* of first-dollar coverage for physician and hospital services but discuss extending publicly funded insurance to cover only catastrophic drug expenditures by patients; it seems that out-of-pocket payments for medically necessary medication below the level of catastrophic somehow differ from payments for the services of the physicians who write the prescriptions. Extending medicare coverage to home care and related services on the same foundation of medical necessity is less straightforward than is the case for drugs. Nonetheless, it remains that for many patients, particularly those with mental illnesses and addictions, home care's admixture of social and health services is precisely what is prescribed for their recovery (Standing Senate Committee 2004).

Another long neglected but critical policy issue relates to productivity — just how efficient and effective are the providers of health services as currently organized and funded? Over the last century, particularly the last 50 years, productivity has increased dramatically in virtually all businesses and industries, including those that provide intensely personal services. The banking/personal finance industry is a case in point. Among the many factors at play (notably, capital investment) is the replacement of human labour by technology, of new technology by old and of low-cost by high-cost labour, the latter made possible through the application both of technology and of new knowledge derived from research.

Hospitals provide a good example of productivity gains in health care. Diagnostic imaging and new, sophisticated laboratory testing have made ambulatory diagnosis an equally if not more important feature of hospitals than inpatient care. Endoscopy, keyhole surgery and many other clinical innovations have replaced interventions that require hospitalization; the new procedures are performed routinely on an "in and out" basis with equally good results and at much less risk and inconvenience to the patient. A compelling argument, backed up by considerable evidence, for net benefits derived from the rapid increase in spending on pharmaceuticals is the fact that the armamentarium of new drugs has allowed for safe and effective outpatient treatment. There is no free lunch, however; a downside of increased out-of-hospital care has been an increased burden on families and communities.

But it is clear that many of those productivity gains in health care have been slow in coming and are far from being fully realized. Much of the use of new imaging technologies, for example, seems to be more additive than substitutive. Patients referred for an MRI scan, for instance, a scarce and expensive resource, will almost certainly have had older diagnostic technologies applied — physical examination, X-ray, ultrasound, CT scan and so forth — all intended to reduce uncertainty about the diagnosis. Public policy and professional guidelines have been slow in developing to help both patients and providers determine the point at which the use of additional diagnostic technologies is just not worth the expense. One of the limits on the productivity of hospital-based surgical facilities in Canada is a shortage of anaesthetists. Why are we not training and deploying nurse anaesthetists, a class of respected health professionals who have worked in hospitals in the United States for many years? The evidence shows that nearly 70 percent of the services billed for by family and general physicians is within the professional competency of nurse practitioners, nurses, counsellors and other lower-cost health professionals (HSRC 1999b). This should tell us something about why we are short of family doctors. Similarly, the evidence shows that fully 20 percent of the work done by overburdened specialists in Ontario falls within the definition of primary care. The long-standing monopoly of the Canadian physician as both gatekeeper and principal provider of publicly insured health care appears, like all monopolies, refractory even to discussion of the kinds of changes that in some countries have already been made. The cost of not proceeding quickly to discussion of and decision on the substitution of health professionals is ruinously high.

Contemporary biomedical and other knowledge related to health care, combined with educational standards, make redefinition of the professional competencies in the whole spectrum of health professions an overdue policy initiative in Canada. But such an initiative will no more be welcomed by the modern-day guilds than it was by the guilds of old. Attacking that issue and the broader policy issue of enhancing productivity in health care will require political courage. It will also require compelling evidence derived from a vastly improved capacity for health information management, especially evidence derived from new measures of the individual and collective benefits of health services of all kinds. But above all it will require an understanding of and commitment to achieving the synergies that can come only from the coordinated and mutually supportive partnership of the full spectrum of providers working within a genuine system.

The latest first ministers' health accords reflect that understanding. Associated with its substantially increased transfers of cash to the provinces and territories for operating purposes, the federal government has earmarked large sums to facilitate policy changes central to system building. There are funds to support the development of consolidated (province-wide) waiting lists based on the acuteness of people's need for services as assessed by standardized, system-wide criteria. There is support for strategies to educate future health professionals in numbers sufficient to meet the country's needs. Funds have been earmarked to accelerate the pace of primary-care reform, including the development of electronic health records, and to speed up development of the capacity for effective health information management generally throughout Canada. Funds have also been designated to extend the principles of medicare to include insurance against catastrophic drug costs, some home-care services and end-of-life care — that is, to make publicly funded health services more comprehensive in scope. The first ministers made particular mention of the importance of developing public health goals, goals presumably antecedent to articulating a vision of what the health care system should be and do for Canadians in the twenty-first century. This is probably the most important policy initiative of all in terms of system building.

The health accords also focus on accountability — measuring and reporting to provincial, territorial and federal taxpayers the benefits of all those billions spent on health care.[3] Accountability is starting to become a real consideration, and it will surely have political consequences. Although the first ministers have been concerned primarily with accountability from an intergovernmental perspective, the question so often posed to Ontario's HSRC — Are we getting our money's worth? — is heard with increasing frequency publicly and in the media, directed particularly at representatives of the provincial and territorial governments, with their prime responsibility for the provision of health services. Credible responses will be imperative as the proportion of provincial spending on health care continues to increase, together with the opportunity cost of diminished support for many other public services, most notably those addressing powerful determinants of poor health such as child poverty, lack of education, unaffordable housing and low income.

With the notable exception of two provinces,[4] both levels of government have signed on to the Health Council of Canada. This new body was created to share information and report on progress made toward implementing the goals and objectives of the accords reached by the first ministers in 2003 and 2004. Its primary purpose is to report to Canadians on how well the system is functioning in terms of optimizing the health of the population and providing individuals with the means to preserve their physical and mental health — to open the "black box" so that the people of every province and territory can see what they are getting for their money. After a halting start attributable to government foot-dragging on its establishment, the council's first report, published early in 2005, gave notice of its intention to set a hectic pace (Health Council of Canada 2005). Reports are promised for later this year on a series of key policy issues: primary health care, home care, pharmaceuticals, health human resources, waiting times and Aboriginal health issues. There is no doubt that other reports will follow on these and many other issues bearing on the council's mandate. The council will also embark on other long-neglected policy initiatives such as hosting a national health human resources summit to identify the impediments to multidisciplinary care. And it will engage the public in discussion of measures to improve accountability for the money spent on health care and on reform — that is, system building.

The provincial governments, for their part, have come to the conclusion that the single funding lever they have used for so many years, powerful as it is, is by itself insufficient to bring about the needed coordination and integration of health care delivery. More and sharper tools are necessary to make a system out of silos. The provinces realize that system building is essential to the achievement of both the greater productivity in health care that accountability requires and the comprehensiveness and continuity of care that their populations demand and deserve. They realize that only governments can pick up the challenge of providing the leadership/governance that is needed to pull together, into systems, the providers of the health services required by their populations, including hospital and physician services.

The approaches vary by province, but Ontario, long the odd man out with respect to regionalization of managerial decision-making in health, exemplifies the accelerated pace of system building, or at least a new focus on "systems thinking." In Ontario, as elsewhere, the main spur to change continues to be financial, although the decline in public confidence that medicare will be "there" for people when they need it is also a vital consideration. The government on whose watch medicare is perceived to fail would suffer the consequence of touching the proverbial third rail; it would surely be destined to spend a good many years in the political wilderness. Despite its imposition of a health levy (thereby breaking a key campaign promise not to raise taxes), the Ontario government is struggling to keep another promise — to balance the budget in its first term. It has not escaped its notice that the share of provincial expenditures on health care is still growing. With the continued application of stringent controls on spending in hospitals and (admittedly less effective) attempts to constrain physician recompense, the rate of increase in the health care budget did slow between 2003 and 2004 (to 5.9 percent), though it still exceeded the rate of inflation and growth in the economy and in government revenues, primarily as a consequence of growing expenditures on pharmaceuticals and home care.

In its report recommending strategies to improve the performance of contributors to an Ontario health care system, the HSRC made two broad policy recommendations:

> adopt a systems view, supported by a comprehensive approach to continuous qualitative improvement, both within the Ministry of Health and externally with the province's health care organizations and providers, which continue to work largely independently of one another

> establish an arm's-length body[5] to advise the minister of health on systems issues and report to the public on health-system performance, which is assessed by means of indicators and measures in five categories: financial, customer satisfaction, internal processes, innovation and improvement, and impact of productivity of the system on the health of the community/population served (HSRC 2000d)

Pursuing the accountability theme and following the commission's recommendation, in 2004 the government of Ontario passed legislation to establish the Ontario Health Quality Council.[6] The responsibilities of the council are to monitor and report to Ontarians on their access to, on the personnel necessary to provide, and on the outcomes of publicly funded health services; it must also support continuous quality improvement in such services. Sensibly, the work of the council is linked with that of the Health Council of Canada through the requirement that they have at least one member in common.

The mandate and presumed modus operandi of the Ontario Health Quality Council will build naturally on those of a provincial pioneer, the Cancer Quality Council of Ontario, which has developed a set of strategy-based system-wide performance indicators to monitor and report to the public on cancer care (Greenberg et al. 2005). The initial report on the quality of cancer care, scheduled for publication in the spring of 2005, will deal with progress toward the achievement of five goals: improved measurement, increased use of evidence, better use of resources, improved access to cancer services and reduction in the burden of cancer.

The work of the Ontario Health Quality Council will also build on the assessment and reporting initiatives of health-service providers themselves. Such initiatives include the Ontario Hospital Association's Balanced Scorecard for Ontario Acute Care Hospitals, practice atlases and other reports by the Institute for Clinical Evaluative Sciences, the Scorecard for Complex Continuing Care and Rehabilitation Hospitals, and other reports that are evolving and increasingly informing the public on many dimensions of the performance of the organizations concerned. It will be up to the Ontario Health Quality Council to integrate these reports so that the government and the public are informed on performance from a systems perspective. So far such reporting is in its infancy, but clearly it is intended to develop and mature rapidly.

A more hotly debated requirement of the legislation is that "health resource providers" (hospitals, nursing homes and homes for the aged, and Community Care Access Centres, or CCACs) enter directly into accountability agreements with the minister of health. The Act also requires the boards of hospitals and other health-service providers to establish performance agreements with their chief executive officers. Based on the principle that "accountability is fundamental to a sound health system," the agreements are sweeping in scope, covering "performance goals and objectives respecting roles and responsibilities, service quality, accessibility of services, related human resources, shared and collective responsibilities for health system outcomes, consumer and population health status, value for money, consistency, and other prescribed matters." Not much is left out!

Although the governance of hospitals and other institutional providers in Ontario remains definitively the responsibility of their boards of directors, the accountability agreements would make explicit the expectation that those boards and their senior managers give priority to the policy directions of a more senior level of governance — the province — of the health care system as a whole. The Act provides the legislative framework for the government to provide, through its minister of health, the system-wide leadership/governance of health services that is the sine qua non of system building.

A second piece of legislation, also passed in 2004, reinforces the theme of accountability of hospitals and other institutional providers of health services.[7] Bill 18 authorizes the Provincial Auditor[8] to examine the financial records of recipients of "reviewable grants" and to report annually to the legislature in the same way that he or she does following examination of the public accounts. This provides for the financial and "value for money" auditing of hospitals, nursing homes, and home-care and mental health agencies — all those organizations that receive government funding. Although focused on financial accountability, this Act, too, constitutes an important tool for fostering the creation of a genuine health-services system in Ontario. At the very least, in support of the concept of "value for money" audits, the *Act Respecting the Provincial Auditor* requires the Ministry of health to be more explicit about the many difficult policy choices that confront hospitals and other institutional care providers, particularly in the face of ongoing revenue constraints. Those choices range from the mundane (Is the nutrition department producing food of good quality at reasonable cost?) to the complex and ethically difficult (Should the expensive and scarce resources of the intensive-care unit be deployed in cases where deployment will likely prove futile?). And they include the perennial but seldom publicly discussed issue of "rates versus numbers" — raising the wages and salaries of employees and other health care providers versus maintaining or increasing their number to support higher-quality care, greater service capacity, building maintenance, capital equipment and so forth. There is no more fundamental (or politically difficult) choice than that!

As for the commission's "adopt a systems view" recommendation, it is increasingly obvious that the ministry's perspective and internal organization are shifting from the traditional departmental or "branch" style to a systems orientation. In the last year or so, policy issues have claimed priority over operational and managerial matters. A clear sign of system building is the creation of an internal Health Results Team, people drawn from within and outside the ministry with a mandate to

> resolve the access-to-services/waiting-time problem
> accelerate the renewal of primary care
> begin developing a system of health information management
> set up the apparatus to foster system building at a local/regional level (devolution) and shift the ministry's focus from micro-management to policy-making and other dimensions of governance

These four thrusts are accompanied by initiatives to strengthen community relations and improve the ministry's external communications. All of this represents a major shift in focus for the Ontario government and its Ministry of Health.

Another sign of system building is the new memorandum of agreement between the government and the Ontario Medical Association.[9] The first page of the agreement states that the Ministry of Health "is charged with the responsibility for health care in the Province of Ontario." With this acknowledgement, Ontario's physicians surely agree that the government must exercise the authority to discharge that responsibility; "he who pays the piper calls the tune" — as it is played by not only physicians but all providers in the system. It will be seen over the next three years how the nonmonetary provisions of this agreement are pursued. The record of follow-up on issues in other agreements of this nature is not encouraging. Nevertheless the 2005 agreement focuses to a remarkable degree on primary-care renewal/reform, the transformation of primary health care from a largely solo, entirely doctor-centric activity providing services to all comers on a fee-for-service basis into a multiprofessional group endeavour providing comprehensive services around the clock to defined populations. This is one of the system-building steps identified as essential by the HSRC more than five years ago. Originally rejected by the OMA's membership during negotiation of the agreement in September 2004, ostensibly on the grounds that it provided too little money for increased rates of recompense for doctors, a focus on transformation of primary health care in Ontario remains a feature of the renegotiated agreement.[10]

With respect to the pace of change, there is no doubt that financial and political circumstances have changed since 1996. The government established and gave the HSRC power to impose change on Ontario's hospitals, and to do so quickly. Clearly, the political risk of restructuring these icons of health care was considered worth bearing given the province's dire financial circumstances. Later, first the Conservative and then the Liberal government made the policy decision to reject the commission's advice to proceed with implementation of primary-care reform over six years in favour of a voluntary, incremental approach. With this decision, the two different approaches to primary care — multidisciplinary teams providing comprehensive services to defined or rostered populations and solo or group practices billing on a fee-for-service basis — will continue side by side. The decision on which approach best suits his or her needs and aspirations will rest with each individual physician. Although much easier from a political perspective than imposing change, running the two models in parallel has a very high cost, to which the renegotiated agreement with the OMA bears witness. It presents the very real risk that the government will have insufficient resources available to provide the generous incentives needed to "buy change" on the scale necessary to create, within a reasonable period, a genuine subsystem of primary care. The decision illustrates both the political power of doctors, acting individually and together, and the government's belief that Ontario's financial circumstances are not as dire as it makes them out to be.

The most encouraging of the system-building initiatives undertaken by the ministry's Health Results Team is that identified explicitly as system integration. After many years of outright opposition to the concept of devolving to regional bodies[11] even limited authority for planning, much less the governance and management of selected health services, Ontario has changed course. It has declared its intention to establish 14 Local Health Integration Networks (LHINs) with the following characteristics and responsibilities.[12]

(1) LHINs will be independent bodies set up under the *Corporations Act*.
(2) Their governance will be by experienced members drawn from the community/region served and appointed by the government (by orders-in- council).
(3) The inaugural CEOs will be appointed by the government and subsequently by each LHIN's board of governors/directors.
(4) LHINs will be categorized as "payers" for health services. Unlike regional health authorities elsewhere, they will not also be "providers." They will not take over or substitute for the governing boards of hospitals or of any other institutional health-service provider.
(5) Their mandates[13] will be to plan, integrate, coordinate and (by 2008) fund some (but not all) of the major contributors to the health care systems they are charged with developing and leading in their communities and regions: "They will provide (the Ministry) with guidelines to policy development, ensure integration takes place in their communities, and generally enable quality and efficient care across the continuum."[14]
(6) The LHINs' authority will be vested in their power to allocate money from an "envelope" provided by the government, in the power to enforce performance agreements made with the providers of health care under their jurisdiction, and potentially in legislation. Absent the direction-setting authority of governance and, until 2008, the power to allocate funds, the LHINs will require resolute and direct support by the minister and the Ministry of Health to establish their bona fides with the spectrum of providers in their regions.
(7) The jurisdiction of each geographically defined LHIN will include family health teams (but not other providers of primary care), hospitals, long-term-care facilities, and CCACs.

The LHINs are being established on a very short timeline. They are expected to begin work in the spring of 2005, the government's having selected board chairs, members and founding chief executive officers. At the outset their roles will probably represent some amalgam of the now-defunct District Health Councils and the regional offices of the Ministry of Health. Their mandates are intended to grow from there, as each LHIN's expertise and experience increases together with the comfort level of the ministry, the region's providers and other stakeholders in working with this important new player.

Another sign that system building has reached the status of "must do" policy is the attention being paid to what the HSRC referred to as the "top priority for building a better health system," health information management (HSRC 1999b). Building on work done by Ontario's Smart Systems for Health since the mid-1990s, the Health Results Team includes a thrust toward finding ways to simplify, consolidate and streamline utilization of existing data sources available to the Ministry of Health. Its responsibilities include developing strategies to rationalize and expand those sources as rapidly as possible in order to access the complete spectrum of data needed to support the effective governance, management and operation of a system of health care that consumes the lion's share of the province's resources. The priority accorded to this key area does not correspond with that recommended by the HSRC, in terms of neither its funding nor its prominence. Nevertheless it is clear that the Ontario government recognizes that the capacity to collect, store, transmit, share, secure, analyze and manage health information is fundamental to the success of all its other health-policy initiatives.

This conclusion is shared by Ottawa and the other provincial/territorial governments. All share in the work of Canada Health Infoway, an independent, arm's-length organization established in 2001 to facilitate partnerships throughout the public and quasi-public sectors of both levels of government in order to foster and accelerate the development of secure, interoperable electronic health-record systems Canada-wide. Now endowed to the tune of $1.1 billion, Canada Health Infoway is engaged in over 50 jointly funded provincial projects across the country, all focused on the development of secure electronic health records incorporating comprehensive information on the diverse interactions between the providers and consumers of health care and the use of those records to enhance care both on-site and at a distance — by "telehealth" (Canada Health Infoway-Inforoute Santé du Canada 2004).[15] All of this work relates to one of six themes, five of which constitute key elements of the electronic health record that sits at the heart of a subsystem of health information management:

> what is referred to as "infostructure," the technology and standards on which an information management system is built and maintained
> "registers" of providers and consumers that ensure the secure identification of participants in health services

> a drug information system to support the electronic prescribing of pharmaceutical agents and the application of relevant clinical guidelines at the point of service
> a diagnostic imaging system to support the transmission, analysis and reporting of X-rays and other such images at a distance
> a laboratory information system to record and report the results of diagnostic tests and to apply relevant clinical guidelines at the point of service
> a public health surveillance system to ensure ready access to the information needed by the health professions to counter threats to public health, such as the SARS experience in Canada

Canada's health care sector has long underinvested in information technology relative to other industries. Canada Health Infoway reports that the average health region's IT budget was just 1.43 percent of its total in 2002, down from 1.88 percent in 2001. Although never announced as policy, here, too, it seems that raising wages and salaries has claimed higher priority than investing in one of the key tools for building and maintaining a sustainable system.

In its report to the government on how to facilitate integration among health care providers at a community level, the HSRC pointed out the value of both removing centrally imposed roadblocks and providing assistance to those "on the ground" eager to achieve greater coordination or integration of their organizations and activities (HSRC 2000a). System building can and should proceed from the bottom up as well as from the top down. Although the government has paid little attention to that HSRC report, an encouraging recent development relating to health information management is the appointment of a chief information officer for a number of Toronto's downtown hospitals. If government policy were in place and widely advertised to encourage and reward such initiatives, system building would proceed much more rapidly everywhere.

It looks like Canada and her provinces and territories are finally determined to organize a genuine system of health care, and perhaps of health *and* health care services — "*the big thing we haven't done yet.*" That's great! But let's hope we can pick up the pace.

NOTES

1 Now approximately 70 percent public and 30 percent private in Canada.
2 Some hospital-based services – for example, long-term and chronic care, some ambulatory services, and private and semiprivate accommodation – are subject to copayment requirements.
3 Estimated by the Health Council of Canada to approach $130 billion in 2004.
4 Alberta and Quebec.
5 Referred to by the HSRC as a Health System Improvement Council.
6 Bill 8: An Act to establish the Ontario Health Quality Council, to enact new legislation concerning health-services accessibility and repeal the Health Care Accessibility Act, to provide for accountability in the health-services sector, and to amend the Health Insurance Act. Royal Assent, June 17, 2004.
7 Bill 18: An Act respecting the Provincial Auditor. Royal Assent, November 20, 2004.
8 Later renamed the Auditor General.
9 Tentatively signed on March 7, 2005.
10 Although the disincentives to remain in fee-for-service practice were reduced.
11 District Health Councils, now defunct, were to *advise* the ministry on local health-planning issues.
12 Online information from the editors of *Healthcare Quarterly,* based on comments by Gail Paech, assistant deputy minister and head of System Integration, Health Results Team, Ministry of Health and Long-Term Care, at an educational conference of the Ontario Hospital Association, February 27, 2005. See also transforminghealth@moh.gov.on.ca
13 Which may later be formalized in legislation.
14 Gail Paech, op. cit.
15 Quebec did not participate in Canada Health Infoway at the outset, but it did starting in 2004.

BIBLIOGRAPHY

Aba, S., W.D. Goodman, and J.M. Mintz. 2002. "Funding Public Provision of Private Health: The Case for a Copayment Contribution through the Tax System." *C.D. Howe Institute Commentary* 163. Toronto: C.D. Howe Institute.

Alberta Health and Wellness. "Health Care Evolution Gains Speed in Alberta." Alberta News Release. January 11, 2005. http://www.health.gov.ab.ca

Barer, Morris. 2005. "Evidence, Interests and Knowledge Translation: Reflections of an Unrepentant Zombie Chaser." *Healthcare Quarterly* 8, no. 1: 46-53.

Barer, Morris, and Greg L. Stoddart. 1991. "Toward Integrated Medical Resource Policies for Canada." Prepared for the federal/provincial/territorial deputy ministers of health.

Birkmeyer, J.D., A.E. Siewers, E.V.A. Finlayson, T. A. Stukel, F.L. Lucas, I. Batista, H.G. Welch, and D.E. Wennberg. 2002. "Hospital Volume and Surgical Mortality in the United States." *New England Journal of Medicine* 346, no. 15: 1128-37.

Birkmeyer, J.D., T.A. Stukel, A.E. Siewers, P.P. Goodney, D.D.E. Wennberg, and F.L. Lucas. 2003. "Surgeon Volume and Operative Mortality in the United States." *New England Journal of Medicine* 349, no. 22: 2117-27.

Canada Health Infoway-Inforoute Santé du Canada. 2004. *2003-2004 Annual Report and Corporate Plan Summary*. Ottawa: Author.

Canadian Institute for Health Information (CIHI). 2001. *Supply, Distribution and Migration of Canadian Physicians, 2000 Report*. Ottawa: Author.

—. 2003. *Health Care in Canada*. Ottawa: Author.

Canadian Institute for Health Information and Statistics Canada. 2004. *Health Care in Canada*. Ottawa: Author.

Chan, Ben. 1999. *Supply of Physicians' Services in Ontario*. Toronto: Institute for Clinical Evaluative Sciences.

—. 2002. *From Perceived Surplus to Perceived Shortage: What Happened to Canada's Physician Workforce in the 1990s?* Toronto: Institute for Clinical Evaluative Sciences.

Commission d'étude sur les services de santé et les services sociaux. 2001. *Report and Recommendations: Emerging Solutions*. Quebec: Ministère de la Santé et des Services Sociaux, Gouvernement du Québec.

"Concern about Future of New Brunswick Physician Supply." 2004. *Health Edition* 8, no 2. www.healthedition.com

Conference Board of Canada. 2004. *Understanding Health Care Cost Drivers and Escalators*. Ottawa: Author. http://www.conferenceboard.ca

Coyte, P., and P. McKeever. 2001. "Home Care in Canada: Passing the Buck." *Canadian Journal of Nursing Research* 33, no. 1: 11-25.

Decter, M. 1994. *Healing Medicare: Managing System Change the Canadian Way*. Toronto: McGilligan.

—. 2000. *Four Strong Winds: Understanding the Growing Challenges to Health Care*. Toronto: Stoddart.

Expert Panel on SARS and Infectious Disease Control. 2004. *For the Public's Health: A Plan of Action, Final Report*. Toronto: Ministry of Health and Long-Term Care.

Finlayson, E.V.A., P.P. Goodney, and J.D. Birkmeyer. 2003. "Hospital Volume and Operative Mortality in Cancer Surgery: A National Study." *Archives of Surgery* 138: 721-6.

Fisher, Elliott S. 2003. "Medical Care: Is More Always Better?" Editorial. *New England Journal of Medicine* 349, no. 17: 1665-7.

Flexner, Abraham. 1910. *Medical Education in the United States and Canada: A Report to the Carnegie Foundation for the Advancement of Teaching.* New York: Carnegie Foundation for the Advancement of Teaching.

Flood, C., and D.G. Sinclair. 2005. "Steering and Rowing in Health Care: The Devolution Option." *Hospital Quarterly* 8, no. 1: 54-7.

Forget, E.L., R.B. Deber, and L.L. Roos. 2002. "Medical Savings Accounts: Will They Reduce Costs?" *Canadian Medical Association Journal* 167, no. 1: 43-7.

Gratzer, D. 1999. *Code Blue: Revising Canada's Health Care System.* Toronto: ECW Press.

Greenberg, A., H. Angus, T. Sullivan, and A.D. Brown. 2005. "Development of a Set of Strategy-Based System-Level Cancer Care Performance Indicators in Ontario, Canada." *International Journal for Quality in Health Care* 17, no. 2: 107-14.

HayGroup. 1999. *Public Behavior, Perceptions and Priorities in the Health Sector: An Overview.* Toronto: Author.

Health Canada. 2001. *Public Home Care Expenditures in Canada, 1975-76 to 1997-98.* Ottawa: Author. Accessed May 26, 2005. http://www.hc-sc.gc.ca/english/care/expenditures/homecare.html

Health Council of Canada. 2005. *Health Care Renewal in Canada: Accelerating Change.* Ottawa: Author.

Health Edition. 2004. "Concern about Future of New Brunswick Physician Supply." *Health Edition* 8, no. 2. www.healthedition.com

Health Services Restructuring Commission (HSRC). 1997a. *A Vision of Ontario's Health Services System.* Toronto: Author.

—. 1997b. "Rebuilding Ontario's Health System: Interim Planning Guidelines and Implementation Strategies – Home Care, Long-Term Care, Mental Health, Rehabilitation and Sub-acute Care." Discussion paper.

—. 1998a. *Change and Transition: Planning Guidelines and Implementation Strategies for Home Care, Long-Term Care, Mental Health, Rehabilitation, and Sub-acute Care.* Toronto: Author.

—. 1998b. "Change and Transition. Planning Guidelines and Implementation Strategies for Home care, Long Term Care, Mental Health, Rehabilitation, and Sub-acute Care." Author: Toronto.

—. 1999a. *Better Hospitals, Better Health Care for the Future: Summary Report on Hospital Restructuring, 1996-1999.* Toronto: Author.

—. 1999b. *Ontario Health Information Management Action Plan: The Top Priority for Building a Better Health System. Advice and Recommendations to the Honorable Elizabeth Witmer, Minister of Health.* Toronto: Author.

—. 1999c. *Primary Health Care Strategy: Advice and Recommendations to the Honorable Elizabeth Witmer, Minister of Health.* Toronto: Author.

—. 1999d. *Proposed Inter-professional Primary Health Care Groups (PCGs) Costing Models: A Technical Costing Report Prepared by Milliman & Robertson, Inc. (Actuaries and Consultants) for the Health Services Restructuring Commission's Primary Health Care Strategy.* Toronto: Author.

—. 2000a. *Advancing Community Integration: Experiences and Next Steps. Advice and Recommendations to the Honourable Elizabeth Witmer, Minister of Health.* Toronto: Author.

—. 2000b. *Looking Back, Looking Forward: A Legacy Report.* Toronto: Author.

—. 2000c. *Seven Points for Action.* Toronto: Author.

—. 2000d. *Strategy for Improving Health System Performance. Advice and Recommendations to the Honourable Elizabeth Witmer, Minister of Health.* Toronto: Author.

Hollander, Marcus, and Neena Chappell. 2002. *Synthesis Report: Final Report of the National Evaluation of the Cost-Effectiveness of Home Care.* Ottawa: Health Transition Fund, Health Canada.

Kent, Tom. 2000. *What Should Be Done about Medicare?* Ottawa: Caledon Institute of Social Policy.

Kizer, K.W. 2003. "The Volume-Outcome Conundrum." *New England Journal of Medicine* 349, no. 22: 2159-61.

Knight, K., ed. 2003. *The Catholic Encyclopedia.* Online ed., vol. 9. Accessed April 14, 2005. www.newadvent.org/cathen/09056a.htm

Lewis, Stephen, and Denise Kouri. 2004. "Regionalization: Making Sense of the Canadian Experience." *Healthcare Papers* 5, no. 1: 12-13.

Lomas, J. 1997. "Devolving Authority for Health Care in Canada's Provinces: Emerging Issues." *Canadian Medical Association Journal* 156: 817-23.

MacKinnon, Janice. 2004. "The Arithmetic of Health Care." *IRPP Policy Matters* 5, no. 3.

Mazankowski, D. 2001. *Premier's Advisory Council on Health for Alberta: A Framework for Reform.* Edmonton: Alberta Health and Wellness.

McEwan, K., and E. Goldner. 2000. *Accountability and Performance Indicators for Mental Health Services and Supports: A Resource Kit Prepared for the Federal/Provincial/Territorial Advisory Network on Mental Health.* Ottawa: Health Canada.

McIntyre, Jane, Tracey O'Sullivan, and Jim Frank. 2003. *Canada's Public Health Care System through to 2020: Challenging Provincial and Territorial Financial Capacity.* Ottawa: Conference Board of Canada.

McKendry, Robert. 1999. *Physicians for Ontario: Too Many? Too Few? For 2000 and Beyond.* Toronto: Ontario Ministry of Health and Long-Term Care.

Metropolitan Toronto District Health Council. 1995. *Directions for Change: Toward a Coordinated Hospital System for Metro Toronto.* Toronto: Author.

Meyer, Christopher, and Stan Davis. 1998. *Blur: The Speed of Change in the Connected Economy.* Reading, MA: Addison-Wesley.

Ontario College of Family Physicians. 1999. *Family Medicine in the 21st Century: A Prescription for Excellence in Health Care.* Toronto: Author.

Ontario Medical Association. 1966. *Primary Care Reform: A Strategy for Stability.* Toronto: Author.

—. Human Resources Committee. 2002. *Position Paper on Physician Workforce Policy and Planning.* April 4. Accessed July 6, 2004. http://www.oma.org/phealth/phr2002.htm

Ontario Ministry of Finance. 1995. *1994-1995 Public Accounts of Ontario: Financial Statements.* Toronto: Author. Accessed June 6, 2005. http://www.gov.on.ca/FIN/english/pacct/1995/95_fse.htm

Ontario Ministry of Health and Long-Term Care. 1988. *Rural and Northern Health: Parameters and Benchmarks Report.* Toronto: Author.

—. 1994. *Putting People First.* Toronto: Author.

—. 1995. *Draft Multi-year Plan Mental Health Reform.* Toronto: Author.

—. 1996. *Rehabilitation Strategy Action Plan.* Toronto: Author.

—. 1997. *The Rural and Northern Health Care Framework.* Toronto: Author.

—. 2002. *The Time Is Now: Themes and Recommendations for Mental Health Reform in Ontario. Final Report of the Provincial Forum of Mental Health Implementation Task Force Chairs.* Toronto: Author.

Picard, André. 1999. "Home Health Care: Only if You Can Afford It." *The Globe and Mail,* December 6.

Prime Minister's National Forum on Health. 1997. *Canada Health Action: Building on the Legacy. Final Report of the National Forum on Health.* PL 090124C. Ottawa: Health Canada Communications.

Provincial Coordinating Committee on Community and Academic Health Science Centre Relations (PCCCAR). 1995a. *New Directions in Primary Health Care.* Toronto: Ontario Ministry of Health and Long-Term Care.

—. 1995b. *Ontario's Academic Health Science Centres: Sustaining Ventures of Their Communities.* Toronto: Ontario Ministry of Health and Long-Term Care.

—. 1997. *Funding Academic Health Science Networks: An Investment in the Future. Part I: The Funding of Postgraduate Medical Education. Part II: The Funding of*

Health Science Research. Toronto: Ontario Ministry of Health and Long-Term Care.

Queen's University School of Policy Studies. 1999. *Path Dependency, Positioning and Legitimacy: Considerations on Public Receptivity to Health Care Reform.* Kingston: School of Policy Studies.

Resource Based Relative Value Schedule Commission (John G. Wade, Chair). 2002. *Report to the Ontario Ministry of Health and Long-Term Care and the Ontario Medical Association.* Vol. 1, *Final Report.* Vol. 2, *Tables.* Toronto: Author.

Rode, M., and M. Rushton. 2002. *Options for Raising Revenue for Health Care.* Discussion paper 9. Ottawa: Royal Commission on the Future of Health Care in Canada.

Royal Commission on the Future of Health Care in Canada. 2002. *Building on Values: The Future of Health Care in Canada.* Ottawa: Author.

Rusk, James. 1996. "Travelling Executioners to Seal Fate of Ontario Hospitals." *The Globe and Mail,* July 15, A3.

Ryten, E. 1997. *Statistical Picture of the Past, Present and Future of Registered Nurses in Canada.* Ottawa: Canadian Nurses Association.

Saskatchewan Health Services Utilization and Research Commission. 1998. "Hospital and Home Case Study." Summary report 10. Saskatoon: Author.

Sinclair, Duncan G. 1966. Speech given to the Annual General Meeting of the Catholic Health Association of Ontario, September 26.

—. 1997. Letter to the Honourable Elizabeth Witmer, Minister of Health. In "Second Quarter Report to the Minister of Health for the Period July 1 - September 30, 1997." Toronto: Health Services Restructuring Commission.

—. 1998. Letter to the Honourable Elizabeth Witmer, Minister of Health. In "Third Quarter Report to the Minister of Health for the Period October 1 - December 31, 1997." Toronto: Health Services Restructuring Commission.

—. 1999-2005. Unpublished speeches. Available on request.

Standing Senate Committee on Social Affairs, Science and Technology. 2002a. *The Health of Canadians: The Federal Role.* Vol. 2, *Current Trends and Future Challenges.* Ottawa: Senate.

—. 2002b. *The Health of Canadians: The Federal Role.* Vol. 6, *Recommendations for Reform.* Ottawa: Senate.

—. 2004. *Mental Health, Mental Illness and Addiction, Interim Reports 1 and 2.* Ottawa: Senate.

Statistics Canada/Canadian Institute for Health Information. 2003. *Health Indicators, 2003.* www.cihi.ca

Thorsell, William. 1998. "Get over It." *Report on Business,* January 10.

Thunder Bay District Health Council. 1994. *Thunder Bay Hospital Services Review – Consolidated Report.* Thunder Bay, ON: Author.

Weissert, W.G. 1992. "Cost-Effectiveness of Home Care." In *Restructuring Canada's Health Services System: How Do We Get There From Here?,* edited by Raisa Deber and Gail G. Thompson. Toronto: University of Toronto Press.

Welch, H.G., D.E. Wennberg, and W.P. Welch. 1996. "The Use of Medicare Home Health Care Services." *New England Journal of Medicine* 335, no. 5: 324-9.

BIOGRAPHICAL NOTES

Peggy Leatt received her university education from the University of Alberta, where she earned a BScN, a master's in health administration (1975) and a Ph.D. in sociology (1980). In 2002 Dr. Leatt joined the faculty at the University of North Carolina at Chapel Hill as a professor in the Department of Health Policy and Administration, School of Public Health. In 2003 she was appointed as chair of the Department of Health Policy and Administration. Prior to joining UNC, Dr. Leatt held the Liberty Health Chair of Health Management Strategies at the University of Toronto. From 1987 to 1998, she was chair of the University of Toronto's Department of Health Administration, Faculty of Medicine. From 1989-98 she was principal investigator of the Hospital Management Research Unit, funded by the Ontario Ministry of Health and Long-Term Care, conducting health systems research in conjunction with providers of health services. From 1998-2000 she was CEO of the Ontario Health Services Restructuring Commission, with the role of designing policies for the reform of the health care system for the province. She cochaired the Blue Ribbon Taskforce for the Association of University Programs in Health Administration and the National Center for Healthcare Leadership in 2004. She has published extensively on topics such as strategic management, health reform, and organizational culture and design. Her current research interests are in the area of patient safety and quality of performance in relation to cancer services.

Mark Rochon has been the president and CEO of the Toronto Rehabilitation Institute since its inception in 1998. In 1996 he became the founding CEO of the Health Services Restructuring Commission. Prior to this he had held senior leadership positions, including president and CEO of Humber Memorial and the Georgetown and District Memorial Hospitals and associate administrator of the Clarke Institute of Psychiatry. He was seconded to the Ministry of Health and Long-Term Care as assistant deputy minister, Institutional Health Group, in 1994. He is chair of the board of the Institute for Work and Health and is a director of the Ontario Hospital Association; he has served as a director of the Ontario Family Health Network. Mark is an assistant professor (status only) in the Department of Health Policy, Management and Evaluation and the Department of Physical

Therapy in the Faculty of Medicine, University of Toronto. He graduated in 1976 with a bachelor of commerce from Queen's University and in 1980 with a master of health sciences (health administration) from the University of Toronto.

Duncan Sinclair, emeritus professor of physiology and fellow of the School of Policy Studies of Queen's University, retired in 1996 as vice-principal (health sciences) and dean of medicine at Queen's. He had served previously in a number of senior administrative roles at Queen's, including vice-principal (institutional relations), vice-principal (services), and dean of arts and science. He chaired Ontario's Health Services Restructuring Commission from 1996 to its sunset in 2000, and following that he served as founding chair and acting CEO of Canada Health Infoway-Inforoute Santé du Canada.